WORKBOOK TO ACCOMPANY
VANDER•SHERMAN•LUCIANO
HUMAN PHYSIOLOGY

WORKBOOK TO ACCOMPANY VANDER•SHERMAN•LUCIANO HUMAN PHYSIOLOGY

Fourth Edition

Matthew J. Kluger
Louis G. D'Alecy

PROFESSORS OF PHYSIOLOGY
THE UNIVERSITY OF MICHIGAN MEDICAL SCHOOL

McGRAW-HILL BOOK COMPANY
NEW YORK ST. LOUIS SAN FRANCISCO AUCKLAND BOGOTÁ HAMBURG
JOHANNESBURG LONDON MADRID MEXICO MONTREAL NEW DELHI PANAMA
PARIS SÃO PAULO SINGAPORE SYDNEY TOKYO TORONTO

Workbook to Accompany Vander, Sherman, and Luciano: HUMAN PHYSIOLOGY

ISBN 0-07-066967-8

2 3 4 5 6 7 8 9 0 HALHAL 8 9 8 7 6

This book was set in Century Schoolbook by Automated Composition Service, Inc.
The editor was Mary Jane Martin;
the cover was designed by Charles A. Carson;
the production supervisor was Charles Hess.
Project supervision was done by The Total Book.
Halliday Lithograph Corporation was printer and binder.

CONTENTS

HOW TO USE THIS WORKBOOK

ORGANIZATION

You will note as you flip through this workbook that there are 20 chapters corresponding to the 20 chapters in the text. Each of these chapters is divided into several modules. Each module should take approximately ½ to 1½ hours to complete. Within each module there are several sections; Objectives, Reading Assignment, Exercises, and Self-Test. Each of these sections is described in full below.

The figures appearing in this workbook are numbered W-1 through W-28. All references to double-numbered figures (8-20, etc.) are figures that appear in Vander, Sherman, and Luciano: *Human Physiology*, fourth edition.

OBJECTIVES

The objectives section of each module contains a listing of the objectives you will be expected to achieve at the end of the module. Read each objective carefully *before* you begin the reading assignment. Concentrate on the portions of the reading that will help you most in completing the objectives. Because educational objectives reflect the aims of a particular course and the value systems of a specific teacher, no one set of objectives meets all requirements. With the assistance of the course director, select from the lists those objectives which meet your needs, modifying them whenever appropriate.

It must be emphasized that the objectives are almost entirely of the cognitive type; few ask the student to manipulate the material extensively or use the information to predict answers to a new problem. This is not because we believe such objectives are unimportant, but rather because explicit answers to such questions are not to be found in the book. We would urge your instructors to add to these objectives additional ones which do tell the student the kinds of manipulations, deductions, predictions, etc., the student should be able to perform.

READING ASSIGNMENT

All reading assignments are from the text *Human Physiology*, fourth edition, by Vander, Sherman, and Luciano.

EXERCISES

When the objectives indicate that a review of materials would be beneficial, exercises have been provided. These exercises may be completed with the help of the text and should be used for review before each test. Each exercise is accompanied by a number in the margin that indicates the page in the text where help in solving the exercise may be found. There is occasionally insufficient space to answer questions in this workbook. Use a separate sheet of paper for those questions requiring long and detailed answers.

SELF-TEST

Each module ends in a self-test. When you feel you can achieve each of the objectives listed for the module, take the self-test. Complete the test at your leisure in a "testing" environment (no books, notes, or distractions). When you have answered as many of the questions as you can, check your answers using the key provided in the back of the questions as you can, check your answers using the key provided. Refer to the pages in your text (shown at the right) for answers that you missed or were unsure about. Remember that the self-test provides only a sample of questions.

ACKNOWLEDGMENTS

The authors thank the staff of the Department of Educational Resource of the School of Dentistry for their assistance in the production of the first edition of this workbook. The experience and training we received greatly facilitated the preparation of this current edition.

Matthew J. Kluger
Louis G. D'Alecy

WORKBOOK TO ACCOMPANY
VANDER•SHERMAN•LUCIANO
HUMAN PHYSIOLOGY

1
A FRAMEWORK FOR HUMAN PHYSIOLOGY

Module I • Mechanism and causality

OBJECTIVES

Upon completion of this module, the student will be able to:

1. Describe the *mechanistic* and *vitalistic* view of life.
2. Define *teleology* and give examples of teleological statements.
3. Define and give an example of *causality* in physiology.
4. Describe why evolution makes it *appear* that most physiological processes are purposeful.

READING ASSIGNMENT

Chap. 1, pp. 1–2.

EXERCISES

PART I

Directions: Below are listed several statements. Describe whether each statement is an example of mechanistic or vitalistic views.

1 The functioning of the brain is the result of millions (perhaps billions) of electro-
1 chemical events.

2 The regulation of blood flow to our brain, kidneys, and other organs is the result
1 of chemical, physical, and spiritual needs.

3 On the basis of our current knowledge of physics and chemistry we cannot thor-
1 oughly explain how the brain stores and retrieves information.

PART II

Directions: Describe why the following statement is teleological. Rewrite the sentence in a way that conveys the information without being an example of teleology.
Statement: During digestion the stomach breaks down food because the body needs
1–2 energy.

SELF-TEST

PART I

Directions: Complete the following items in the space provided.

1 The view that forces beyond chemistry and physics are part of living organisms is called ______________________.

2 The explanation of events in terms of purpose is known as ______________.

3 The ______________________ view of life holds that all living processes are ultimately understandable in terms of physical and chemical laws.

4 The reason so many physiological processes appear to be purposeful is because of millions of years of ______________________ selecting for those processes that have ______________________.

PART II

Directions: Circle the correct answer(s).

1 The functioning of any organ system can ultimately be explained in terms of chemical and physical laws. This viewpoint is
a mechanistic. b teleological. c vitalistic.

2 The heart pumps proportionately more blood to the kidneys than to some other organ because the kidney needs to remove a tremendous amount of waste products from the blood. This statement is an example of
a mechanism. b teleology. c vitalism.

3 The reason most bodily activities appear to be purposeful is because
a teleology is a powerful force.
b mechanism is sufficient to describe most biological processes.
c evolutionary processes result in the maintenance of responses having survival value.

Module II • A society of cells

OBJECTIVES

Upon completion of this module, the student will be able to:

1 Define *cells*.
2 List the fundamental activities common to virtually all cells.
3 State that the differences in cell function generally are attributable to specializations of one or more of the fundamental common properties of cells.
4 Define *cell differentiation*.
5 List the four categories of differentiated cells as (a) muscle cells, (b) nerve cells, (c) epithelial cells, and (d) connective-tissue cells.
6 Describe the general characteristics of the four categories of differentiated cell types.
7 Define *tissues*.
8 List the four general classes of tissues as (a) muscle tissue, (b) nerve tissue, (c) epithelial tissue, and (d) connective tissue.

9 Differentiate between the "formal" and the "commonly used" definition of tissues.
10 Define *organ* as a collection of tissues joined in a structural unit to serve a common function.
11 Define *organ system*.
12 List the 10 organ systems and describe their primary function.

READING ASSIGNMENT

Chap. 1, pp. 2–5.

EXERCISES

PART I

Directions: Answer the following questions in the space provided.

2 1 List the four categories of differentiated cells and describe the general types of functions each perform.

4–5 2 Define tissues, organs, and organ systems.

4 3 Distinguish between the technical and the more common definition of tissues.

5 4 List the organ systems of the body and describe their functions.

SELF-TEST

PART I

Directions: Complete the following items in the space provided.

1 ______________________ is the process by which the initially identical cells present during the earliest stages of development not only undergo anatomical alteration but also acquire specialized functional properties.

2 ______________________ cells generate force and produce motion.

3 ______________________ cells cover the surfaces of the body or individual organs or line the walls of various tubular and hollow structures within the body.

4 ______________________ cells generate electric signals and have the ability to send these signals from one area of the body to another.

5 The major function of ______________________ cells is to anchor and support the structures of the body.

6 Four similarities among virtually all cells are ______________________,

______________________, ______________________,

and ______________________.

PART II

Directions: Circle the correct answer(s).

1 The four general categories of tissues are:
  - a connective tissue
  - b liver tissue
  - c nerve tissue
  - d heart tissue
  - e muscle tissue
  - f epithelial tissue

2 The following are examples of organ systems:
  - a digestive
  - b adrenal
  - c heart
  - d nervous
  - e respiratory

PART III

Directions: Circle T for true and F for false.

T F 1 A cell from the human body and one from a unicellular organism are identical.

T F 2 The primary function of the circulatory system is to regulate the plasma composition through execretion of organic wastes, salts, and water.

T F 3 The immune system is responsible for support, protection, and movement of the body.

T F 4 Muscle, nerve, epithelial, and connective-tissue cells constitute the four general categories of differentiated cells.

T F 5 The primary functions of the respiratory system are to exchange the gases oxygen and carbon dioxide and to regulate hydrogen-ion concentration.

T F 6 The primary function of the endocrine system is to protect against injury and dehydration and to regulate body temperature.

Module III • The internal environment and general principles

OBJECTIVES

Upon completion of this module, the student will be able to:

1 Define *internal environment* and *external environment.*
2 Define *extracellular fluid.*
3 Identify Claude Bernard as being the first person to clearly describe the importance of the maintenance of a relatively constant internal environment.
4 Identify, by volume (liters) and by percent, approximately how much body water is divided between intracellular and extracellular compartments in a "70-kg man."
5 Identify, by volume and by percent, approximately how much extracellular fluid is divided between interstitial fluid and plasma in a "70-kg man."
6 Describe the general concept of *control* in physiological systems.
7 Identify which systems are involved in the transmission and integration of information.

READING ASSIGNMENT

Chap. 1, pp. 6–9.

EXERCISES

PART I

8 Directions: Fill in the missing labels and values in Fig. W-1.

PART II

Directions: Answer the following questions in the space provided.

1 Explain what is meant by the internal environment. Why do you think that Claude Bernard's idea concerning the "fixity of the internal environment" has been called
7 the "single most important unifying idea" in physiology?

____

____

____

9 2 Explain what is meant by control in physiology.

____

____

____

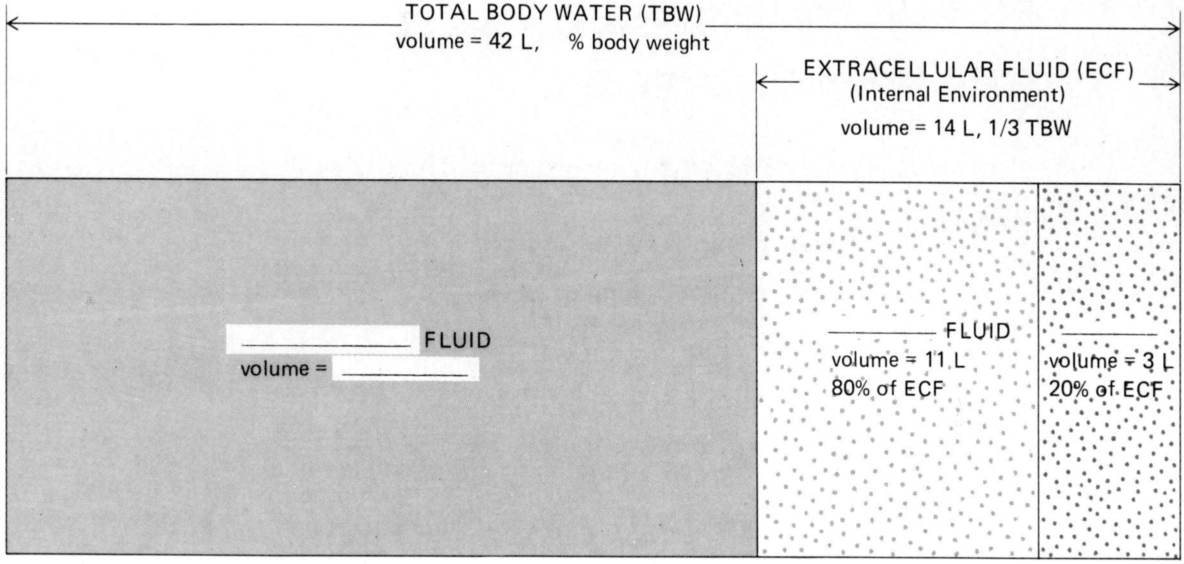

Fig. W-1: Fluid compartments of the body.

SELF-TEST

PART I

Directions: Complete the following items in the space provided.

1 The body's internal environment is the ________________________ that bathes each of the body's cells.

2 The extracellular fluid is divided between ________________________ and ________________________.

3 The transmission and integration of information is performed primarily by the ________________________ and ________________________ systems.

PART II

Directions: Circle the correct answer(s).

1 In the "standard" 70-kg man, interstitial fluid volume is approximately
a 10% of ECF. b 50% of ECF. c 80% of ECF. d equal to ECF.

2 In the "standard" 70-kg man, plasma volume is approximately
a 1 L. b 2 L. c 3 L. d 4 L.

3 In the "standard" 70-kg man, intracellular fluid volume is approximately
a $\frac{1}{3}$ of TBW. b $\frac{2}{3}$ of TBW. c equal to TBW.

4 In the "standard" 70-kg man, extracellular fluid volume is approximately
a 5 L. b 9 L. c 14 L. d 18 L.

Answers

CHAPTER 1 • MODULE I

PART I

1 vitalism (1)
2 teleology (1)
3 mechanistic (1)
4 evolution, survival value (2)

PART II

1 a (1)
2 b (1–2)
3 c (3)

CHAPTER 1 • MODULE II

PART I

1 differentiation (2)
2 muscle (2)
3 epithelial (4)
4 nerve (4)
5 connective tissue (4)
6 they exchange material with their immediate environment, obtain energy from organic nutrients, synthesize complex proteins, duplicate themselves (2)

PART II

1 a, c, e, f (4)
2 a, d, e (5)

PART III

1 F (2)
2 F (5)
3 F (5)
4 T (2)
5 T (5)
6 F (5)

CHAPTER 1 • MODULE III

PART I

1 extracellular fluid (7)
2 interstitial fluid, plasma (8)
3 nervous, endocrine (9)

PART II

1 c (8)
2 c (8)
3 b (8)
4 c (8)

2
CELL STRUCTURE

Module I • Cell structure

Module I • Cell structure

OBJECTIVES

Upon completion of this module, the student will be able to:

1 Define *metabolism.*
2 Define *cell organelles.*
3 List the approximate sizes of the cell organelles shown in Fig. 2-1, p. 14.
4 State the size of the smallest object clearly seen by the human eye, the light microscope, and the electron microscope.
5 Distinguish between *cytoplasm* and *cytosol.*
6 List the major cell organelles.
7 Describe the general structure and function of the following:
   a plasma membrane
   b nucleus, including nuclear envelope, nuclear pores, nucleolus, chromatin, and chromosomes
   c endoplasmic reticulum (contrast the functions of granular and agranular ER)
   d ribosomes (contrast the functions of free and bound)
   e Golgi apparatus
   f secretory vesicles
   g mitochondria, including cristae and internal space or matrix
   h lysosomes
   i peroxisomes
8 Define *cytoskeleton.*
9 List four classes of filaments that make up the cell's cytoskeleton as a. microfilaments, b. intermediate filaments, c. muscle thick filaments, and d. microtubules.
10 List the protein subunits for microfilaments, muscle thick filaments, and microtubules.
11 Describe the function of each of the classes of filaments.

READING ASSIGNMENT

Chap. 2, pp. 13–23.

EXERCISES

PART I

Directions: For each of the following organelles, state if it is bounded by a membrane or is nonmembranous and describe its function.

21 1 lysosomes

20 2 Golgi apparatus

15 3 nucleus

18–19 4 ribosomes

18–19 5 endoplasmic reticulum

20 6 mitochondria

7 peroxisomes 22

____

____

____

8 microtubules 22–23

____

____

____

PART II

Directions: Contrast the functions of granular with agranular endoplasmic reticulum 18–19

____

____

____

PART III

Directions: Fill in the following table.

Filaments	Protein Subunits	
microtubules	______________	22
______________	myosin	
microfilaments	______________	
______________	several proteins	

SELF-TEST

PART I

Directions: Circle the correct answer(s).

1 Most cell organelles
   a are located in the nucleus.
   b are suspended in a fluid known as interstitial fluid.
   c are enclosed by membranes.

2 The nucleus
   a is surrounded by two membranes called the nuclear envelope.
   b has openings into the cytoplasm known as nuclear pores.
   c contains the nucleolus, the site of assembly of lysosomes.
   d has chromosomes containing the molecules of DNA.

3 Granular (rough surfaced) endoplasmic reticulum
  a is a nonmembranous structure.
  b has ribosomes embedded in its surface.
  c transports proteins synthesized by ribosomes.
  d contains enzymes for the synthesis of fats.

4 Mitochondria
  a are found in the nucleus.
  b are surrounded by a single membrane known as cristae.
  c are the primary site of ATP production.
  d are involved in digestion of complex substances such as bacteria and cellular debris engulfed by the cell.

5 Nonmembranous intracellual structures include
  a ribosomes. b filaments. c lysosomes. d mitochondria.

PART II

Directions: Match the term in Column A with the characteristic in Column B by placing the appropriate letter on the line.

	Column A	Column B
1.	_______ microtubules	a. composed of actin
2.	_______ muscle thick filaments	b. composed of myosin
3.	_______ microfilaments	c. composed of tubulin
4.	_______ intermediate filaments	d. composed of several proteins

Answers

CHAPTER 1 • MODULE I

PART I

1 c	(15)
2 a, b, d	(15–18)
3 b, c	(18–19)
4 c	(20–21)
5 a, b	(18)

PART II

1 c	(22)
2 b	(22)
3 a	(22)
4 d	(22)

3
CHEMICAL COMPOSITION OF THE BODY

Module I • Atoms and molecules
Module II • Structure and properties of organic molecules

Module I • Atoms and molecules

OBJECTIVES

Upon completion of this module, the student will be able to:

1 Define *chemical element.*
2 Describe the structure of an atom by identifying the location within the atom of the subatomic particles—*electrons, protons,* and *neutrons.*
3 Describe the relative *mass* and *electric charge* of each subatomic particle and the atom as a whole.
4 Define *atomic number* and differentiate it from *atomic weight.*
5 Differentiate between *gram-atomic weight* and *mole.*
6 List the four atoms that account for 99 percent of the atoms in the body.
7 List the seven major minerals and the 13 trace elements that are essential for maintaining the structure and function of the body.
8 Describe the role of *covalent* and *double bond* in the formation of *molecules.*
9 Describe the formation of *ions* and *polar molecules* by differentiating between the process of ionization and the uneven distribution of charge within a molecule.
10 Differentiate between *anions* and *cations.*
11 Define electrolyte.
12 Differentiate between *polar* and *nonpolar* molecules.
13 Describe the role of the *hydrogen bond* in maintaining the liquid state.
14 Define and give the general formula for the *hydrolytic reaction.*

15 Define *solute, solvent,* and *concentration.*
16 Define *ionic bond.*
17 Differentiate between *polar* and *nonpolar solvents* and describe their role in determining the solubility of polar and nonpolar solutes.
18 Describe the relationship between *amphipathic* molecules and *micelles* and state their importance in the body.
19 Define *molecular weight, mole,* and *molar.*
20 Define *acid* and *base.*
21 Distinguish between a weak acid and a strong acid.
22 Distinguish between *acidic* and *alkaline* solutions.
23 Define pH and describe the effect of changes in hydrogen ion concentration on pH.

READING ASSIGNMENT

Chap. 3, pp. 24–34.

EXERCISES

PART I

Directions: Answer the following questions in the space provided.

30–32 1 Describe the properties water has that make it an excellent solvent for many types of molecules.

____

____

____

33 2 Define pH and state the difference between a strong acid and a weak acid.

____

____

____

27–30 3 Describe the difference between an ion and a polar molecule.

____

____

____

4 List the major elements in the body and four of the major minerals. 26

____

____

____

PART II

Directions: Complete the following items in the space provided.

1 All the atoms of a specific type are known as specific ____________________ ________. 24

2 The three subatomic particles are ____________________, ____________________, and ____________________. 25

3 A strong chemical bond is formed when ____________________ are shared to produce a covalent bond. 27

4 Ions and molecules with a number of ionized groups, when dissolved in ____________________, can conduct electricity and are often referred to as ____________________. 28–29

5 The loss of an electron results in the formation of a ____________________ charged ion. 28

6 ____________________ have a positive and ____________________ have a negative charge. 28

7 The atomic weight is the relative weight of an atom and is proportional to the sum of the number of ____________________ and ____________________ that the atom contains. 25

8 ____________________ is responsible for water being in the liquid state over a wide range of temperatures. 30

9 Acids are molecules that give rise to ____________________ ions. 33

10 Polar solvents will tend to dissolve ____________________ molecules, and ____________________ solvents will tend to dissolve nonpolar molecules. 32

11 Amphipathic molecules form ____________________ when mixed with water. 32

12 One ____________________ of a compound dissolved in one ____________________ of solution produces a 1 *M* solution. 33

13 As the hydrogen-ion concentration of a solution increases the pH of the solution

34 ________________________.

PART III

Directions: Match the items in Column A with the characteristics in Column B by placing the appropriate letter on the line.

Column A

1 ______ hydrogen, oxygen, carbon, and nitrogen 26

2 ______ water 30

3 ______ hydrogen ion 33

4 ______ carbon 27

5 ______ amphipathic molecule 32

Column B

a its concentration determines the acidity of a solution.
b is a polar solvent.
c can form four chemical bonds.
d accounts for 99 percent of the atoms in the body
e contain both polar and nonpolar regions.

SELF-TEST

PART I

Directions: Circle T for true and F for false.

T F 1 All molecules in the body can easily dissolve in water.
T F 2 A proton and electron are the same weight but opposite in charge.
T F 3 The presence of hydrogen in a molecule makes it an acid.
T F 4 Water is a polar molecule.
T F 5 Virtually all 90 natural chemical elements are required for maintaining the structure and function of the body.
T F 6 The pH increases as the hydrogen-ion concentration decreases.
T F 7 Only ionized molecules can go into solution.
T F 8 Most molecules in the body are in greater than 1 *M* concentration.

PART II

Directions: Complete the following items in the space provided.

1 ________________________ is the principle solvent in the body.

2 The ________________________ of a solution is a measure of the concentration of hydrogen ions in solution.

3 ________________________ are formed by linking atoms together.

4 A(n) ________________________ is positively charged if it contains fewer ________________________ than protons.

5 A 1 *M* solution of glucose contains the same number of ________________ __________ as a 1 *M* solution of sucrose.

6 Molecules with ionized groups and ions form an ________________________ ________ when dissolved in water.

7 A(n) ________________________________ bond is formed when two atoms share an electron.

PART III

Directions: Circle the correct answer(s).

1 Solutions
  a have a liquid component called the solvent.
  b are formed when a solute dissolves in the solvent.
  c containing large numbers of hydrogen ions are acidic.
  d of nonpolar molecules form ions in water.
  e in nonpolar solvents do not contain ions.

2 The 24 chemical elements essential in the body
  a are present in equal amounts.
  b are all in the ionized form.
  c can be synthesized by the body.
  d form both polar and nonpolar molecules.
  e form both the solute and solvents in the body.

3 Water
  a is the most numerous molecule in the body.
  b is a polar solvent.
  c is the solvent for both ions and many organic molecules.
  d can mix with some polar molecules when the polar molecules form micelles.
  e is formed by a very strong bond between hydrogen and oxygen.

4 The pH of a solution
  a is the negative logarithm to the base 10 of the hydrogen ion concentration.
  b above 7 is said to be alkaline.
  c below 7 is said to be acidic.
  d increases as the hydrogen-ion concentration decreases.
  e is changed by both organic and inorganic molecules.

Module II • Structure and properties of organic molecules

OBJECTIVES

Upon completion of this module, the student will be able to:

1 Define and differentiate among *inorganic chemistry, organic chemistry,* and *biochemistry.*

2 Define *polymer*.
3 Describe the general characteristics of the chemical bonds formed by the carbon atom.
4 List the four major categories and their subclasses of organic molecules in the body and the characteristics of each as presented in Table 3-5, p. 35.
5 Define *monosaccharide, disaccharide,* and *polysaccharide* and give examples of each of these types of carbohydrates.
6 List the three subclasses of lipids and give the distinguishing characteristics of each.
7 Distinguish between an *amino acid* and an *amino acid side chain* as subunits of protein.
8 Define *amino acid, peptide bond, polypeptide, alpha helix, oligomeric proteins,* and *protomer.*
9 Distinguish among *primary, secondary, tertiary,* and *quartenary* structure of proteins.
10 Differentiate and give examples of covalent, ionic, hydrogen, and van der Waals bonding in determining the three-dimensional shape of proteins.
11 Identify the two types of *nucleic acids* and state the role of each in the synthesis of proteins.
12 Describe the three major differences between *RNA* and *DNA*.
13 Define *glycolipid, lipoprotein,* and *nucleoprotein.*

READING ASSIGNMENT

Chap. 3, pp. 34–47.

EXERCISES

PART I

Directions: Answer the following questions in the space provided.

1 For each of the following major categories of organic molecules, list the major subclasses and provide their characteristics.

a carbohydrates ____________________

35 ____________________

b lipids ____________________

35 ____________________

c proteins ____________________

35 ____________________

d nucleic acids ____________________

35 ____________________

2 Describe the factors that determine a protein's tertiary structure.

____

____

____ 41–42

PART II

Directions: Complete the following items in the space provided.

1 ______________________ are formed by linking together smaller organic molecular subunits. 34

2 The four major categories of organic molecules in the body are ______________, ______________, ______________, and ______________. 34

3 ______________________ provide cells with energy and are readily soluble in water. 34–36

4 ______________________ are insoluble in water and can be used by most cells to provide energy. 35

5 The ______________________ bond links amino acids together to form polymers that are the ______________________ structure of protein molecules. 38–39

6 ______________________, ______________________, and ______________________ are bonding forces that contribute to the tertiary structure of protein. 44

PART III

Directions: Match the item in Column A with the characteristic in Column B by placing the appropriate letter on the line.

	Column A	Column B
38	1 _______ protein	a reserve fuel
44	2 _______ DNA	b short chain of amino acids
36	3 _______ lipid	c stores genetic information
36	4 _______ phospholipid	d sex hormones
41	5 _______ alpha helix	e major source of nitrogen
38	6 _______ steroids	f number and type of amino acids in a sequence
39	7 _______ primary protein structure	g membrane structure

34 8 ______ glucose — h six-carbon molecule

44 9 ______ RNA — i secondary protein structure

39 10 ______ peptide — j decodes genetic information

SELF-TEST

PART I

Directions: Complete the following items in the space provided.

1 When a molecule of fatty acid contains no double bonds, it is said to be ______________________.

2 The term used to refer to the class of molecules formed when all three hydroxyls in glycerol are substituted with fatty acids is ______________________.

3 Inorganic chemistry is the chemistry of ______________________.

4 A branch of organic chemistry related specifically to living substances is ______________________.

5 The liver can link many glucose units together to form glycogen, which is classed as a(n) ______________________.

6 Sugars composed of two other sugars joined together are called ______________________.

7 The breakdown of carbohydrates to CO_2 and H_2O serves what function? ______________________

____

____

PART II

Directions: Circle the correct answer(s).

1 A peptide bond occurs between which two functional groups?
a carboxyl and hydroxyl
b amino and hydroxyl
c two amino groups
d amino and carboxyl

2 The primary structure of proteins refers to the
a interaction of more than one peptide chain.
b alpha helix configuration.
c sequence of amino acids.
d random coiling prior to alpha helix formation.

3 Which of the following can be considered an organic compound?
a sodium chloride
b carbohydrates
c calcium phosphate
d hydrochloric acid

4 Which of the following describe the role(s) of protein in the body? Proteins
   a provide most of the chemical energy for the cells.
   b account for 50% of the organic material in the body.
   c catalyze most chemical reactions in the body.
   d are necessary for energy storage.

5 Which of the following is the best reason why an entire field of chemistry is devoted to the study of carbon compounds? Carbon is
   a the most abundant atom in nature.
   b the only atom used by human cells.
   c able to form four separate bonds with other atoms.
   d unable to form bonds with other carbon atoms.

6 The body's most important monosaccharide is
   a galatose. b lactose. c glucose. d sucrose.

7 Common plant polysaccharides include
   a starch. b cellulose. c glycogen. d glucose.

8 Which of the following compose the basic components of a neutral fat molecule?
   a amino acids b fatty acids c glucose d ethanol e glycerol

9 Some hormones and cholesterol are common examples of
   a phopholipids. b proteins c steroids d fatty acids.

10 Because they contain both a polar and a nonpolar end, effective for water lipid interfaces, one of the following groups is a major component of cell membranes. Which one?
   a phospholipids b fatty acids c proteins d carbohydrates

PART III

Directions: The illustrations labeled A through E in Fig. W-2 are examples of the complete or partial structures of different classes of compounds. Match them with their correct names in the column below.

1 ______ neutral fat

2 ______ protein

3 ______ steroid

4 ______ phospholipid

5 ______ carbohydrate

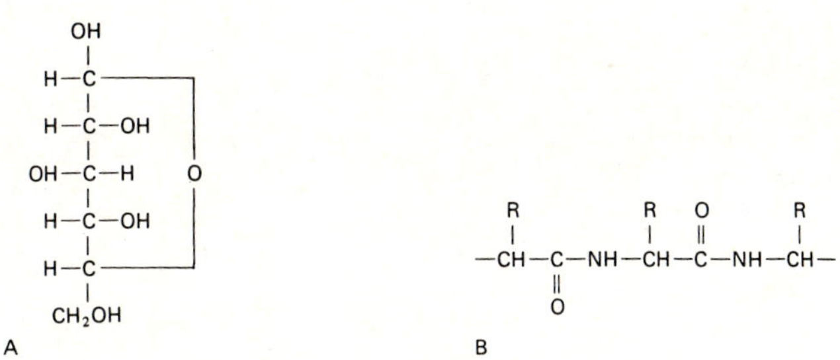

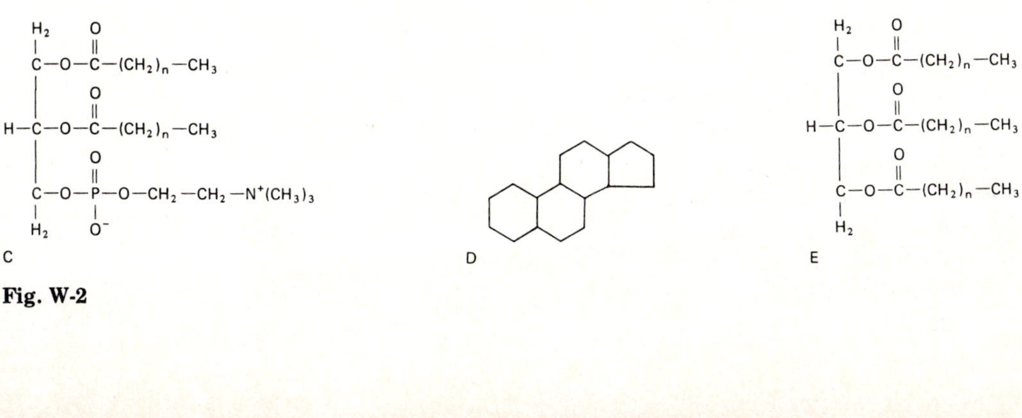

Fig. W-2

PART IV

Directions: Match the terms in Column A with the correct chemical group shown in Column B.

Column A	Column B
1 ______ amino	a OH
2 ______ phosphate	b NH_2
3 ______ hydroxyl	c COOH
4 ______ carboxyl	d PO_4

Answers

CHAPTER 3 • MODULE I

PART I

1 F	(32)
2 F	(25)
3 F	(33)
4 T	(30)
5 F	(26)
6 T	(33–34)
7 F	(32)
8 F	(33)

PART II

1 water	(30)
2 acidity or pH	(33)
3 molecules	(26)
4 ion; electrons	(28)
5 molecules	(33)
6 electrolyte	(28–29)
7 covalent	(27)

PART III

1 a, b, c, e	(31–33)
2 d, e	(26, 30–31)
3 a, b, c, d	(30–32)
4 a, b, c, d, e	(33–34)

CHAPTER 3 • MODULE II

PART I

1 saturated	(37)
2 neutral fats or triacylglycerols	(36)
3 noncarbon molecules	(34)
4 biochemistry	(34)
5 polysaccharide	(35)
6 disaccharides	(35)
7 provides major source of energy	(35)

PART II

1 d	(38)
2 c	(39)
3 b	(34)
4 b, c	(38)
5 c	(34)
6 c	(34)
7 a, b	(35)
8 b, e	(36)
9 c	(38)
10 a	(35)

PART III

1 E	(37)
2 B	(39)
3 D	(38)
4 C	(37)
5 A	(36)

PART IV

1 b	(40)
2 d	(37)
3 a	(40)
4 c	(40)

4

MOLECULAR CONTROL MECHANISMS—DNA AND PROTEINS

Module I • Protein binding sites
Module II • Genetic information and protein synthesis
Module III • Cell division and differentiation; mutation; cancer; recombinant DNA

Module I • Protein binding sites

OBJECTIVES

Upon completion of this module, the student will be able to:

1 Define *ligand, chemical specificity, affinity, saturation,* and *competition.*
2 Describe the characteristics of protein binding sites using the terms ligand, chemical specificity, affinity, saturation, and competition.
3 Describe the roles that electric charge and shape of the binding site and ligand have in protein–ligand interactions.
4 Distinguish between chemical specificity and affinity (both high and low).
5 Describe the roles of free ligand concentration and the binding site affinity in determining the degree of saturation of a binding site.
6 Describe the role of competition between natural ligands and drugs in determining the effects of the drugs.
7 Describe the process of protein aggregation; describe the role *aggregation factors* have in embryonic growth.
8 Define *catalyst, enzyme, substrates*, and *product.*

9 Describe the importance enzymes have in biological systems.
10 Describe the basis for the selective action of hormones.
11 Describe the role protein binding sites have in the detection of chemical messengers (both intracellular and extracellular).
12 List temperature and acidity as nonspecific factors that can alter protein shape.
13 Define and describe *allosteric modulation* using the terms functional site, regulatory site, modulator molecules, and conformational changes.
14 Define and describe *covalent modulation.*
15 Describe the role of protein kinase in the phosphorylation, and phosphoprotein phosphatase in the dephosphorylation of proteins.

READING ASSIGNMENT

Chap. 4, pp. 48–58.

EXERCISES

PART I

Directions: Answer the following questions about Fig. W-3 in the space provided.

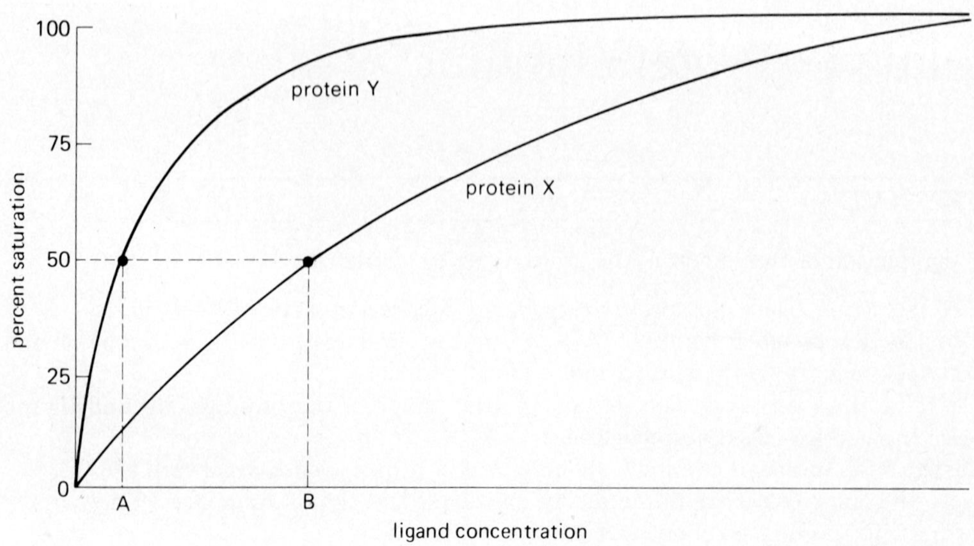

Fig. W-3

1 Which protein (X or Y) has the higher binding affinity for the ligand? ______

2 What could explain the above differences in binding affinities? 50–53

____

____

____

3 How could a modulator substance alter the shapes of curves for proteins X and Y? 56–58

____

____

____

PART II

Directions: Define the following terms.

1 ligand ______________________________

______________________________ 49

2 binding site ______________________________

______________________________ 49

3 competition ______________________________

______________________________ 53–54

4 aggregation factors ______________________________

______________________________ 54–55

5 enzymes ______________________________

______________________________ 54

6 substrates ______________________________

______________________________ 54–55

7 allosteric modulation ______________________________

______________________________ 56

8 covalent modulation ______________________________

______________________________ 57

PART III

Directions: Contrast the role of protein kinase and phosphoprotein phosphatase in the process of protein phosphorylation and dephosphorylation.

____

____

______________________________ 58

SELF-TEST

PART I

Directions: Complete the following items in the space provided.

1 A ________________ is any molecule or ion that can bind to the surface of another molecule by forces other than covalent bonds.

2 The chemical specificity of a protein binding site is determined by the ________________ of the protein molecule.

3 Binding sites that bind a ligand weakly are called ________________.

4 When all the binding sites of a protein are occupied, the binding sites are said to be fully ________________.

5 Many drugs produce their effects by competing with the body's natural ligands for ________________.

6 The proper alignment of cells during embryonic development is assisted by plasma membrane proteins containing specific binding sites known as ________________.

7 Protein substances that accelerate chemical reactions but do not themselves undergo any net chemical change during the reaction are known as ________________.

8 Ligands that bind to enzymes' binding sites are known as ________________, and the molecules that are ultimately formed from these ligands are known as ________________.

9 Allosteric modulation involves changing the ________________ of the binding site protein molecules.

10 The enzyme phosphoprotein phosphatase results in the ________________ of proteins.

PART II

Directions: Circle the correct answer(s).

1 When two ligands, X and Y, are able to bind to the same binding sites, the amount bound to that binding site is dependent on
a the concentration of each ligand.
b the relative affinities of the binding sites for each ligand.

2 The following are capable of altering a protein's binding sites:
a pH
b temperature

c allosteric modulators
d protein kinase in the presence of ATP.

3 In altering enzymatic activity, modulators
a bind with the enzyme functional binding site.
b change the shape of the functional binding site.
c bind to the protein at the regulatory site.
d always increase the activity of the enzyme.

4 The probability that a given binding site will be occupied by a ligand depends on
a the affinity of the binding site for the ligand.
b the concentration of free ligand in the solution.
c the presence or absence of other ligands with similar properties.
d the presence or absence of modulators.

5 Which of the following statements are correct concerning altering protein shape?
a Phosphorylation of a protein always increases the affinity of the functional site.
b The enzyme protein kinase catalyzes the transfer of phosphate from a protein to ATP.
c the phosphorylation of a protein results in allosteric modulation.
d The enzyme phosphoprotein phosphatase results in the removal of the phosphate group from the phosphorylated protein.

Module II • Genetic information and protein synthesis

OBJECTIVES

Upon completion of this module, the student will be able to:

1 Define *DNA, gene, RNA, nucleotide, base, double helix, triplet code, termination code words,* and *messenger RNA.*
2 State the location of protein synthesis.
3 Define *transcription* and *translation.*
4 State the differences between DNA and RNA.
5 Describe *base pairing.*
6 Describe the function of *RNA polymerase* and its dependence on DNA.
7 Describe the function of the *promoter* and the termination sequence in mRNA synthesis.
8 Describe *RNA processing* by stating the relationship of *codons, termination codons, exons,* and *introns* to the final stage of transcription.
9 Describe the interaction of mRNA, ribosomes, ribosomal RNA (rRNA), and transfer RNA (tRNA) in protein assembly.

10 Describe the role of the *nucleolus* in protein synthesis.
11 Define *anticodon.*
12 Define *polyribosome.*
13 Describe the posttranslational processing of proteins.
14 Summarize the four events of transcription (see Table 4-1, p. 68).
15 Summarize the nine events of translation (see Table 4-1, pp. 68–69).
16 Describe induction and repression of protein synthesis.
17 Describe the control of mRNA synthesis in terms of the *operon, repressor protein, operator gene,* and *inducing molecule.*

READING ASSIGNMENT

Chap. 4, pp. 58–72.

EXERCISES

PART I

Directions: Answer the following questions.

1 List the sequence of events leading from DNA to protein synthesis as outlined in Table 4-1, pp. 68–69.
transcription:

____

____

____

translation:

____

____

____

69–70 2 Describe the process of induction and repression in regulating protein synthesis.

____

____

____

PART II

Directions: Define the following terms.

1 nucleotide ______________________________

44 ______________________________

2 transcription ____

____ 60

3 translation ____

____ 60

4 promoter ____

____ 62

5 termination sequence ____

____ 62

6 codon ____

____ 62

7 exons ____

____ 62

8 introns ____

____ 62

9 anticodon ____

____ 66

10 operon ____

____ 70

11 repressor protein ____

____ 70

SELF-TEST

PART I

Directions: Complete the following items in the space provided.

1 The portion of a DNA molecule containing the information required to determine the amino acid sequence of a single polypeptide chain is known as a ____________ ____________________.

2 Each nucleotide of DNA contains one of four bases—____________________ ____________, ____________________, ____________________ ____________, and ____________________.

3 The transfer of the genetic message from DNA to RNA is called ______________; the assembly of the proper sequence of amino acids to form a protein is called ______________.

4 The various tRNAs, with their specific amino acid, base-pair through their ______________ with the corresponding ______________ in mRNA.

5 A number of ribosomes may be attached to the same strand of mRNA forming ______________.

PART II

Directions: Circle the correct answer(s).

1 Ribonucleic acid (RNA)
  a is the basic carrier of genetic information from cell to cell.
  b is a protein.
  c is composed entirely of the same nucleotides found in DNA.
  d can transfer information from DNA in the nucleus to the site of protein synthesis.

2 Most protein synthesis occurs in the
  a nucleus.
  b nucleolus.
  c cytoplasm.
  d mitochondria.
  e extracellular fluid.

3. Which of the following identify differences between DNA and RNA?
  a number of strands in a molecule
  b base composition
  c sugar composition
  d number of different bases in a single molecule
  e types of chemical linkage between bases

4 The genetic code for DNA includes which of the following?
  a only four bases
  b codons composed of four base sequences
  c potentially 64 codons
  d some base sequence that do not code for a specific amino acid
  e some base sequence that code for more than one amino acid

5 Which of the following is (are) true of RNA?
  a When DNA unwinds in the synthesis of mRNA, only one of the two DNA chains is used to form a single mirror-image chain of mRNA.
  b The formation of mRNA does not involve making a mirror image of the entire DNA molecule.
  c DNA codon C-G-T becomes mRNA codon G-C-A.
  d DNA codon G-C-A becomes mRNA codon C-G-T.

6 Choose the proper order for the following sequence of events leading from DNA to protein synthesis:
  (1) Elongation of protein chain.

(2) mRNA passes from the nucleus to the cytoplasm where one end of the mRNA molecule binds to a ribosome.
(3) Free amino acids combine with their corresponding tRNAs.
(4) Transcription of DNA to mRNA.
(5) The three base anticodons in tRNA pair with the corresponding codons in mRNA attached to the ribosomes.
(6) Termination of protein chain.

a 1, 2, 3, 4, 5, 6
b 4, 6, 2, 1, 3, 5
c 3, 6, 2, 5, 1, 4
d 2, 5, 4, 6, 1, 3
e 4, 2, 3, 5, 1, 6

7 The process of a DNA molecule splitting and the pairing of free nucleotides with the bases of each DNA strand to give rise to two new molecules of DNA containing one new and one old strand is best named

a transcription.
b reverse transcription.
c replication.
d differentiation.

Module III • Cell division and differentiation; mutation; cancer; recombinant DNA

OBJECTIVES

Upon completion of this module, the student will be able to:

1 Describe the process of DNA *replication.*
2 Describe the process of cell division using the terms *interphase, chromatin, chromatids, histones, centromere, spindle apparatus, centrioles, mitosis*, and *cytokinesis.*
3 Define *cell differentiation* and describe how it occurs.
4 Define *mutation.*
5 List the major environmental factors that increase the rate of mutations.
6 List three general effects mutations may have on a cell.
7 Define the term *inborn error of metabolism.*
8 Define natural selection and describe the process by which it occurs.
9 State the major abnormalities of cancer cells.
10 Define *malignant tumor, metastasis, carcinogen*, and *oncogene.*
11 Describe the role *restriction nucleases* and *ligases* have in formation of recombinant DNA.

12 Describe the potential long-range benefits and hazards of recombinant DNA technology.

READING ASSIGNMENT

Chap. 4, pp. 72–79.

EXERCISES

PART I

Directions: Answer the following questions in the space provided.

77 1 "Since most mutations are harmful, it would be best if mutations never occurred." Do you agree with this statement? Why?

78 2 Describe the role of restriction nucleases and ligases in the formation of recombinant DNA.

PART II

Directions: Define the following terms.

1 interphase

73

2 histones

73

3 mitosis

73

4 cytokinesis

73

5 mutation

75

6 inborn errors of metabolism ______________________________

______________________________ 77

7 oncogene ______________________________

______________________________ 78

SELF-TEST

PART I

Directions: Complete the following items in the space provided.

1 The period between the end of one cell division and the beginning of the next is called ______________________________.

2 Any alteration in the genetic message carried by DNA is called a(n) ______________________________.

3 Two general properties of cancer cells are ______________________________ and ______________________________.

4 A restriction nuclease splits molecules of ______________________________ into a number of smaller fragments.

5 When recombinant DNA is inserted into a living cell, both sets of genes may be transcribed into mRNA and translated into ______________________________.

PART II

Directions: Circle the correct answer(s).

1 Which of the following statements are true concerning the process of cell division?
   a Most cells spend most of their time in the interphase period of cell division.
   b When DNA threads have been duplicated during early cell division, they are joined together over a small segment of their length in a region known as the centriole.
   c Just prior to cell division, the duplicated DNA-protein threads (chromatin) become highly coiled and condense to form structures called centromeres.
   d The process of nuclear division leading to the separation of identical sets of chromosomes is called mitosis.
   e The spindle fibers of the spindle apparatus act as if they are pulling the chromosome segments toward the poles of the cell during division.

2 Which of the following are major environmental factors that increase the rate of mutations?
   a atomic radiation
   b sunlight
   c x-rays
   d cosmic rays
   e certain chemicals
   f reading physiology texts

3 Which of the following are true of natural selection?
 a It is not affected by mutations.
 b It may result in a sturdier, more effective organism.
 c It generally occurs slowly over long periods of time.
 d It has little effect on the survival rate of organisms.
 e Small changes that are beneficial (given enough time) can produce large changes in the structure and function of an organism.

4 The control of mRNA synthesis is achieved by a repression-induction process. Which of the following form a part of this control?
 a A repressor gene contains the coded information for the synthesis of a repressor protein.
 b A repressor protein is synthesized in the standard way via a repressor gene.
 c The repressor protein may combine with the initial gene of an operon known as the operator gene.
 d The repressor gene is part of a DNA molecule.
 e The combination of the repressor protein with the operator gene prevents synthesis of the operon's mRNA.
 f The induction process occurs when an inducer molecule combines with the repressor protein, thereby inactivating the repressor.

Answers

CHAPTER 4 • MODULE I

PART I

1 ligand (49)
2 shape (49)
3 low-affinity sites (51)
4 saturated (51)
5 binding sites (54)
6 aggregation factors (54)
7 enzymes (54)
8 substrates, products (54–55)
9 shape (56)
10 dephosphorylation (58)

PART II

1 a, b (53–54)
2 a, b, c, d (56–57)
3 b, c (56)
4 a, b, c, d (49–57)
5 d (56–58)

CHAPTER 4 • MODULE II

PART I

1 gene (58)
2 adenine, thymine, guanine, cytosine (59)
3 transcription; translation (60)
4 anticodon; codon (66)
5 polyribosomes (67)

PART II

1 d (58)
2 c (58)
3 a, b, c (60)
4 a, c, d, e (59)
5 a, b, c (remember, uracil replaces thymine in RNA) (60–61)
6 e (68–69))
7 c (70–71)

CHAPTER 4 • MODULE III

PART I

1 interphase (73)
2 mutation (75)
3 uncontrolled growth, loss of specialized cell functions (77)
4 DNA (78)
5 proteins (78)

PART II

1 a, d, e (73)
2 a, b, c, d, e (76)
3 b, c, e (77)
4 a, b, c, d, e, f (70)

5

ENERGY AND CELLULAR METABOLISM

Module I • Energy and determinants of biochemical reaction rates
Module II • ATP and cellular energy transfer
Module III • Carbohydrate, fat, and protein metabolism, and vitamins

Module I • Energy and determinants of biochemical reaction rates

OBJECTIVES

Upon completion of this module, the student will be able to:

1 Define *metabolism, catabolism, anabolism,* and *dynamic steady state.*
2 Define *energy, law of conservation of energy, kinetic* and *potential energy, chemical energy,* and *calorie.*
3 Describe the role of *activation energy* in chemical reactions.
4 Describe the effect of temperature on the rate of chemical reactions.
5 List the determinants of biochemical reaction rates as (a) temperature, (b) molecular concentrations, and (c) concentration of enzymes.
6 Describe and give examples of the law of mass action.
7 State the three basic characteristics of catalysts.
8 Describe the mechanism of enzyme action, including the concept of active or binding sites and chemical specificity.
9 Describe the role of *cofactors* (both metal ions and coenzymes) in biochemical reactions.
10 Describe the role of vitamins in biochemical reactions.
11 List the three major factors influencing the rate of enzyme-mediated reactions.

12 Describe the roles that enzyme induction and enzyme repression have in enzyme-mediated reactions.
13 Describe the role *allosteric* and *covalent modulation* have in enzyme-mediated reactions.
14 Describe the roles rate-limiting reactions or enzymes have in metabolic pathways.
15 Describe the role of end-product inhibition in metabolic pathways.
16 Describe the difference between reversible and irreversible chemical reactions.

READING ASSIGNMENT

Chap. 5, pp. 80–89.

EXERCISES

PART I

Directions: Answer the following items in the space provided.

81 1 What is the difference between potential and kinetic energy?

82 2 How does the magnitude of the activation energy for a given reaction affect that reaction?

82–83 3 List the factors affecting biochemical reactions rates. Why is temperature generally not of major significance?

84 4 Describe why changes in substrate concentration, enzyme concentration, and enzyme activity affect the rate of enzyme-mediated reactions.

5 Describe the role of allosteric and covalent modulation in enzyme activity. **89 and Chap. 4, pp. 56–58**

____

____

____

6 What determines whether a biochemical reaction is reversible or irreversible? **88**

____

____

____

PART II

Directions: Define the following terms.

1 catabolism ______________________________

______________________________ **80**

2 anabolism ______________________________

______________________________ **80**

3 calorie ______________________________

______________________________ **81**

4 enzymes ______________________________

______________________________ **83**

5 cofactors ______________________________

______________________________ **85**

6 coenzymes ______________________________

______________________________ **85**

7 rate-limiting reactions ______________________________

______________________________ **87**

8 end-product inhibition ______________________________

______________________________ **87**

SELF-TEST

PART I

Directions: Complete the following items in the space provided.

1 When the rates of chemical synthesis and degradation are in balance in biological systems, this is called dynamic ______________________________.

2 Reactions that result in the fragmentation of a molecule into smaller parts are called ____________________; those reactions that lead to the production of larger organic molecules are called ____________________.

3 The hotter an object is the faster its molecules move and the greater is the molecule's ____________________ energy.

4 To upset the balance of forces in a molecule, a quantity of energy known as ____________________ must be added.

5 Three factors that affect the rates of biochemical reactions are ____________________, ____________________, and ____________________.

6 Organic cofactors are termed ____________________.

7 The organic portion of coenzyme molecules are derived from ____________________.

8 The rates of enzyme-mediated reactions are dependent on ____________________, ____________________, and ____________________.

9 Spontaneously ____________________ (*reversible* or *irreversible*) reactions release large quantities of energy.

10 Reversible reactions involve ____________________ exchanges of energy.

PART II

Directions: Circle the correct answer(s).

1 Rates of biochemical reactions vary with
  a temperature.
  b magnitude of activation energy.
  c concentration of enzymes.
  d concentration of reactants.
  e activation of enzyme molecules.

2 Which of the following are examples of the law of mass action when considering the reaction A + B = X + Y? A, B, X, and Y are all equal concentrations at equilibrium.
  a Addition of A causes an increase in X and Y.
  b Addition of A causes an increase in X but does not affect the concentration of Y.
  c Addition of A increases the concentration of A, B, X, and Y.
  d Addition of A results in a reduction in the concentration of B.
  e Addition of A will affect only the concentration of A.

3 Adding heat to a chemical reaction
  a increases the kinetic energy of molecules.
  b increases the rate of molecular motion.

c slows down molecules so they react better.
d increases the frequency of molecular collisions.

4 Which of the following statements are true concerning enzyme-mediated reactions?
a Increasing the concentration of substrate will, by mass action, increase the rate of the reaction.
b Through enzyme induction, certain enzymes have increased synthesis when substrate is available.
c Through enzyme repression, the accumulation of product molecules can turn off the synthesis of the enzyme responsible for forming the product.
d The concentration of cofactors can directly affect the activity of enzymes and, therefore, the rate of the reaction.
e Modulator molecules can bind to allosteric enzymes, thereby resulting in a change in the rate of the reaction.

Module II • ATP and cellular energy transfer

OBJECTIVES

Upon completion of this module, the student will be able to:

1 Describe the role of adenosine triphosphate (ATP) in cellular metabolism.
2 State the amount of energy released by hydrolysis of ATP to ADP + P_i.
3 Distinguish between *substrate phosphorylation* and *oxidative phosphorylation*.
4 Describe the role of coenzymes in the breakdown of carbohydrates, fats, and proteins.
5 Define *cytochromes;* describe the role cytochromes have in oxidative phosphorylation.
6 Contrast the location of oxidative phosphorylation with substrate phosphorylation.
7 Identify the role of oxygen in oxidative phosphorylation; know the overall reaction of oxidative phosphorylation as: coenzyme–2H + $\frac{1}{2}$ O_2 in the presence of cytochromes yields coenzyme + H_2O + 52 kcal/mol.
8 Contrast the function of *peroxisomes* with that of mitochondria.
9 Identify the source of most of the hydrogen atoms in oxidative phosphorylation (or the citric acid or tricarboxylic acid cycle).
10 Diagram the Krebs cycle pathway by listing where acetyl coenzyme A enters the cycle, where carbon dioxide is formed, and where hydrogen atoms are formed, and the seven intermediates in the cycle.

11 State the total amount of ATP formed directly in the Krebs cycle and by the oxidative phosphorylation of each 2-carbon fragment entering the cycle.
12 Define *glycolysis.*
13 Distinguish between *anaerobic* and *aerobic* conditions.
14 List the types of fuel that can be used in glycolysis and in the Krebs cycle.
15 Identify the location of glycolysis within the cell.
16 List the 11 reactions of glycolysis in appropriate order.
17 List which reactions in glycolysis require ATP and which generate ATP.
18 Outline the net chemical transformation in glycolysis as: glucose + 2ADP + $2P_i$ yields 2 lactic acid + 2ATP + $2H_2O$.
19 Identify the reactions in glycolysis during which phosphate is added to "glucose" from ATP and those during which phosphate is transferred to ATP.
20 Describe the ultimate fate of glucose metabolism when oxygen is present and when oxygen is absent.
21 Describe three conditions in which glycolysis plays a major role in ATP generation.

READING ASSIGNMENT

Chap. 5, pp. 89–97.

EXERCISES

PART I

Directions: Fill in the blank spaces.

89 1 ADP + P_i + ____________ kcal/mol→ ATP + ____________.

2 Coenzyme-2H + ____________ in the presence of ____________

90 ____________ → coenzyme + H_2O + 52 ____________ /mol.

3 The net reaction for glycolysis is glucose + ____________ ADP + 2

____________ → ____________ +

95 ____________ ATP + ____________ H_2O.

4 In the Krebs cycle, acetyl coenzyme A—1→ citric acid—2→ ____________

____________ —3→ ____________ —4→ ____________

____________ —5→ ____________ —6→ ____________

94 ____________ —7→ ____________.

PART II

Directions: Answer the following items in the space provided.

1 Identify the reaction steps in the Krebs cycle where hydrogen atoms are transferred to coenzyme carrier molecules. **94**

____

____

____

2 Beginning with glucose, list the 11 reactions in glycolysis. **96**
a Which reactions require energy in the form of ATP?
b Which reactions generate energy in the form of ATP?

____

____

____

____

3 Describe the difference between the Krebs cycle and oxidative phosphorylation including site and reactions. **92–94**

____

____

____

4 Describe three special cases in which glycolysis provides most, and in some cases all, of a cell's ATP. **97**

____

____

____

SELF-TEST

PART I

Directions: Complete the following items in the space provided:

1 Most ATP synthesis within cells occurs in the ____________________

________ by the process of ____________________.

2 When ATP is converted to ADP, ________ kcal/mol of energy is released.

3 By passing through the ____________________ chain, energy is released in the mitochondria in small efficient steps rather than all at once.

4 Various intermediates derived from the breakdown of ______________________

__________, ______________________________, and ____________________

____________________ can enter the Krebs cycle.

5 In the absence of oxygen the end product of glucose metabolism is ____________

____________________.

6 When oxygen is present, the end products of glucose metabolism are __________

______________________ and ______________________________.

7 Other names for the Krebs cycle are the ______________________________

or ______________________________.

8 In the Krebs cycle hydrogen is transferred to coenzyme carrier molecules at the following reactions:

isocitric acid to ______________________________

______________________________ to succinic acid

succinic acid to ______________________________

malic acid to ______________________________.

9 In the glycolytic pathway, glucose —1→ ______________________________

—2→ ______________________________ —3→ ______________________________

—4→ ______________________________ —5→ ______________________________

—6→ ______________________________ —7→ ______________________________

—8→ ______________________________ —9→ ______________________________

—10→ ______________________________ —11→ lactic acid or ______________

____________________ when oxygen is present.

PART II

Directions: Circle the correct answer(s).

1 Oxidative phosphorylation
   a permits an efficient recovery of energy from substrates.
   b cannot proceed without oxygen.
   c takes place in mitochondria.
   d permits approximately 40 percent energy recovery.
   e regenerates coenzyme for another cycle.

2 Glycolysis in the absence of oxygen
   a can begin with carbohydrate, lipid, or protein.
   b results in the net gain of 2 ATP/mol of glucose.
   c leads to the formation of pyruvic acid as its end product.
   d occurs in the cytosol of the cell.

3 In the overall chemical transformation in glycolysis
   a 2 molecules of lactic acid are formed for every molecule of glucose.
   b there is a net gain of 2 molecules of ADP for every molecule of glucose consumed.
   c water is formed.
   d oxygen is consumed.

4 Combining the reactions of the Krebs cycle and oxidative phosphorylation, for every 2-carbon fragment that enters the mitochondria
   a 12 molecules of ATP are formed.
   b 2 molecules of carbon dioxide are formed.
   c 1 molecule of lactic acid is formed.
   d 2 molecules of oxygen are consumed.

Module III • Carbohydrate, fat, and protein metabolism, and vitamins

OBJECTIVES

Upon completion of this module, the student will be able to:

1 List the total amount of energy stored in glucose and the actual amount of energy transferred to ATP during glycolysis, during the Krebs cycle, and during oxidative phosphorylation.
2 Describe the chemical structure, function, and primary storage sites of glycogen.
3 Describe the synthesis and breakdown of glycogen as outlined in Fig. 5-15 (p. 100).
4 Describe the pathways involved in glucose synthesis as diagramed in Fig. 5-16, (p. 101); state which reactions are irreversible.
5 Describe where protein, lactic acid, and glycerol can enter the glucose synthetic pathway.
6 List the approximate total body content (energy/g) and total body energy stores (in kcal and in percent) of triacylglycerols, proteins, and carbohydrates.
7 Define and state the function of *adipocytes* and *adipose tissue.*
8 Describe the metabolism of triacylglycerols as outlined in Fig. 5-17 (p. 103).
9 Describe the synthesis of fatty acids.
10 State why glucose can be converted to fat, but the fatty acid portion of fat cannot be converted to glucose.
11 Define *protease.*
12 Outline the two types of reactions—oxidative deamination and transamination—by which the amino group is removed from amino acids.
13 Identify the nitrogen-containing end products of protein metabolism.
14 Describe the pathway for synthesis of amino acids as outlined in Fig. 5-19 (p. 106).

15 Define *essential amino acid.*
16 Describe the interconversions of carbohydrates, fats, and proteins as outlined in Fig. 5-21 (p. 108), highlighting the reversible and irreversible reactions.
17 Define *essential nutrient.*
18 Distinguish between *growth factors* and *vitamins.*
19 List the water- and fat-soluble vitamins; describe the general role of the water- and fat-soluble vitamins.

READING ASSIGNMENT

Chap. 5, pp. 97–109.

EXERCISES

PART I

Directions: Answer the following questions in the space provided.

1 When oxygen is present, approximately how much energy is released from the catabolism of glucose? How much of this energy is lost as heat and how much is stored as ATP? What is the difference in ATP production when oxygen is either
99 present or absent?

____

____

____

100–101 2 Describe which reactions in the glycolytic pathway are irreversible.

____

____

____

3 Fill in the following chart of the fuel content of an *obese* person:

	Total Body Content (kg)	Energy per Gram (kcal/g)	Total Energy (kcal)	Content (%)
Triacylglycerols	25.0			
Proteins	9.5			
Carbohydrates	1.0			

102

104 4 Describe why fatty acids cannot be used to synthesize new glucose.

____

5 Diagram an oxidative deamination and a transamination of an amino acid. **105**

6 Describe the advantage of storing fuels in the form of fat rather than as carbohydrate. **104**

7 Describe the difference between a growth factor and a vitamin. **109**

PART II

Directions: Define the following terms.

1 adipocyte ______ **102**

2 protease ______ **104**

3 essential amino acid ______ **107**

4 essential nutrient ______ **108**

SELF-TEST

PART I

Directions: Complete the following items in the space provided.

1 In the absence of oxygen only ______ molecules of ATP can be formed by glycolysis per molecule of glucose.

2 Most glycogen is stored in ________________________________.

3 Glycogen is synthesized from ________________________________.

4 Triacylglycerols are formed by combining three ________________________________

with ________________________________.

5 In ________________________________ the amino group is released as a molecule of ammonia and replaced by an oxygen atom to form a keto acid.

6 In ________________________________ there is a transfer of the amino group from an amino acid to a keto acid.

7 Two molecules of ammonia are linked with carbon dioxide to form ____________

________________________ in the liver.

8 Amino acids that cannot be produced by the body are called ________________

________________.

9 Fatty acids cannot be converted into glucose because of the irreversibility of the

pyruvic acid-to-________________________________ reaction.

10 The ________________________________-soluble vitamins function as coenzymes.

PART II

Directions: Circle the correct answer(s).

1 Which of the following statements are true concerning the energy yield from glucose?
   a The total amount of chemical energy that is stored in glucose is 266 kcal/mol.
   b When oxygen is available, the net yield of ATP from glucose is 38 ATP/mol of glucose.
   c In the absence of oxygen the net yield of ATP from glucose is 2 ATP/mol of glucose.
   d The overall efficiency of the conversion of glucose to energy in the cell when oxygen is available is approximately 39 percent.
   e In the absence of oxygen this efficiency rises to 61 percent.

2 Concerning the interconversion of carbohydrate, fat, and protein
   a all three classes can enter the Krebs cycle through some intermediate.
   b glucose can be converted into fat or amino acids.
   c fatty acids can be converted into glucose.
   d amino acids can be converted to fat.
   e amino acids can be converted to other amino acids by oxidative deamination.

Answers

CHAPTER 5 • MODULE I

PART I

1 steady state (80)
2 catabolic reactions; anabolic reactions (80)
3 kinetic (81)
4 activation energy (82)
5 temperature, molecular concentrations, presence of enzymes (83)
6 coenzymes (85)
7 vitamins (85)
8 substrate and product concentration, enzyme concentration, enzyme activity (85)
9 irreversible (88)
10 small (88)

PART II

1 a, b, c, d, e (82–85)
2 a, d (83)
3 a, b, d (81–82)
4 a, b, c, d, e (85–87)

CHAPTER 5 • MODULE II

PART I

1 mitochondria, oxidative phosphorylation (90)
2 7 (89)
3 cytochrome (91)
4 proteins, carbohydrates, fats (92)
5 lactic acid (97)
6 carbon dioxide, water (97)
7 citric acid cycle, tricarboxylic acid cycle (92)
8 alpha ketoglutaric acid; alpha ketoglutaric acid, fumaric acid; oxalacetic acid (94)
9 1. glucose 6-phosphate; 2. fructose 6-phosphate; 3. fructose 1,6-diphosphate; 4. dihydroxyacetone or 3-phosphoglyceraldehyde; 5. 3-phosphoglyceraldehyde; 6. 1,3-diphosphoglycerate; 7. 3-phosphoglyceric acid; 8. 2-phosphoglyceric acid; 9. phosphoenolpyruvate; 10. pyruvic acid; 11. carbon dioxide and water. (96–97)

PART II

1 a, b, c, d, e (90–91)
2 b, d (95)
3 a, c (95)
4 a, b, d (93)

CHAPTER 5 • MODULE III

PART I

1 two (99)
2 skeletal muscle and liver (100)
3 glucose (100)
4 fatty acids; glycerol (102)
5 oxidative deamination (105)
6 transamination (105)
7 urea (106)
8 essential amino acids (107)
9 acetyl coenzyme A (101, 104)
10 water (109)

PART II

1 b, c, d (99)
2 a, b, d (108)

6

MOVEMENT OF MOLECULES ACROSS CELL MEMBRANES

Module I • The cell membrane structure, and diffusion
Module II • Mediated-transport systems, and osmosis
Module III • Endocytosis, exocytosis, membrane junctions, epithelial transport, and glands

Module I • The cell membrane structure, and diffusion

OBJECTIVES

Upon completion of this module, the student will be able to:

1. Differentiate between the *plasma membrane* and the nonspecific membranes found throughout the cell.
2. Describe two general categories of cell function that are provided by membranes in terms of *selective permeability* and *specific binding sites.*
3. Define *peripheral proteins* and *integral proteins* in plasma membranes.
4. Describe the *fluid-mosaic model* of plasma membranes by identifying the structural and functional role played by phospholipids, cholesterol, peripheral proteins, and integral proteins in plasma membranes.
5. Define *diffusion.*
6. Define and describe the relationships among *concentration gradient, net flux,* and *diffusion equilibrium.*
7. List the factors that affect the rate of diffusion.
8. Describe why large organisms cannot rely entirely on diffusion to move molecules.
9. Define membrane *permeability constant* (or coefficient).
10. Describe the effect of concentration gradient, molecular weight, chemical structure, and temperature on the rate of diffusion and on the membrane permeability constant.
11. Differentiate between molecules that diffuse through the lipid bilayer portion of the membrane and those that diffuse through protein channels.

12 Define *membrane potential* and *electrochemical gradient* and their effect on ionic flux across membranes.
13 Describe how alterations in the structure and composition of a membrane regulate membrane permeability.

READING ASSIGNMENT

Chap. 6, pp. 110–120.

EXERCISES

PART I

Directions: Answer the following questions in the space provided.

1 Label and describe the function of each component of the plasma membrane indicated in Fig. W-4

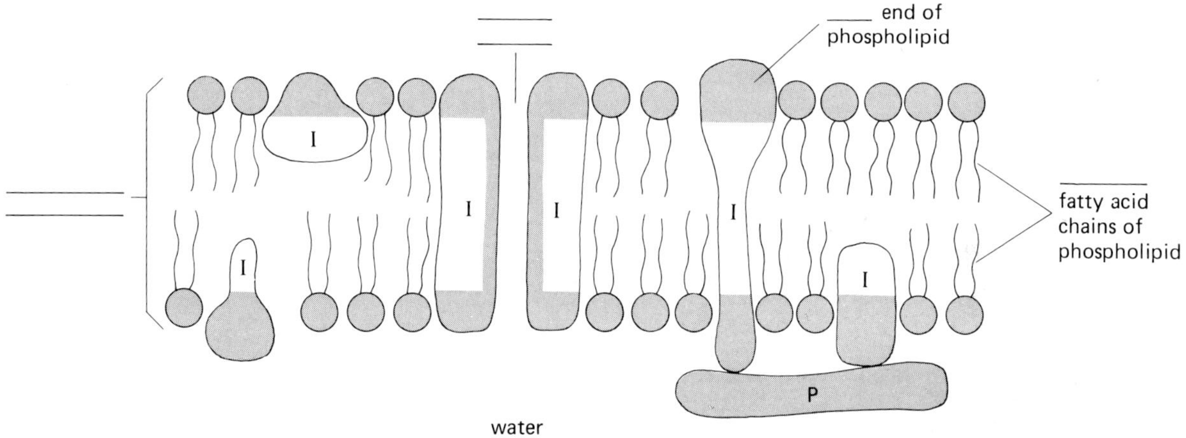

Fig. W-4

In Fig. W-4 I designates ______________________ and P designates ______________________. **113**

2 Discuss the functional advantages of a nonhomogeneous plasma membrane. **118–120**

____

____

____

3 Describe the contribution of membrane potential to the movement of polar versus nonpolar molecules across a cell membrane. **120**

____

____

____

PART II

Directions: Complete the following items in the space provided.

1 The ____________________ separates the cell contents from extra-
110 cellular medium.

2 The two general contributions of membranes to cell function are ____________
110 ____________ and ____________________.

3 Most membranes comprise a bimolecular ____________________
111 matrix in which ____________________ are embedded.

4 ____________________ is the movement of molecules from one lo-
114 cation to another by ____________________ molecular motion.

5 The difference between two one-way fluxes is known as ____________
117 ________.

6 The rate of diffusion depends on the ____________________ and
the ____________________ of the molecule and on the nature of
116 the solution.

7 The rate of diffusion across membranes is a thousand to a million times
____________________ (larger/smaller) than diffusion of the same
118 molecule in water.

8 ____________________-soluble molecules rapidly diffuse through
119 the lipid portion of the membrane.

9 ____________________ molecules diffuse across cell membranes
119 more slowly than do lipid-soluble substances.

10 Membrane permeability can be regulated by alterations in the ____________
120 ____________ and ____________________ of the membrane.

PART III

Directions: Answer the following questions in the space provided.

113 1 Draw a cross section of a typical cell membrane and label each component.

2 List the factors that affect diffusion in a membrane-free solution. **116–117**

____

____

____

3 List the factors that affect the membrane permeability coefficient. **118**

____

____

____

4 List three substances that diffuse through lipid bilayers. **119**

____

____

____

5 List three substances that diffuse through protein channels. **119**

____

____

____

SELF-TEST

PART I

Directions: Circle T for true and F for false.

T F 1 The surface of the cell contains almost all the membrane structure of the cell.

T F 2 The membrane permeability coefficient of a cell does not change once the cell is mature.

T F 3 The only important function of membranes is to serve as selective barriers to the diffusion of molecules.

T F 4 One-way flux is another name for net diffusion.

T F 5 Fatty acids and steroids diffuse through the lipid portion of the membrane.

T F 6 Integral proteins can be removed from cell membranes by washing the membrane in water.

T F 7 Membrane proteins can alter the barrier function and the scaffolding function of the plasma membrane.

T F 8 At diffusion equilibrium there is no further net change in concentration of the two compartments.

T F 9 The permeability of the membrane is altered by changes in the protein pathway or in the pores.

T F 10 Integral proteins are not involved in plasma membrane permeability changes.

PART II

Directions: Circle the correct answer(s).

1 When a cell has reached diffusion equilibrium with its surrounding environment, the following conditions exist.
  a There is no random movement of particles.
  b Molecules are still moving in both directions across the membrane.
  c The pores in the membranes close.
  d There can be large fluxes but no net flux across the membrane.
  e The permeability of the membrane reaches its lowest point.

2 The membrane permeability coefficient is altered by
  a temperature.
  b lipid solubility.
  c pore size.
  d membrane protein configurations.
  e molecular size and charge.

Module II • Mediated-transport systems, and osmosis

OBJECTIVES

Upon completion of this module, the student will be able to:

1 Define *carrier* and describe its role in *mediated transport;* distinguish between mediated transport and diffusion.
2 List the three steps in membrane translocation by mediated transport.
3 Describe the properties of specificity and saturation as they relate to protein binding sites and the carrier hypothesis.
4 Define and differentiate between *facilitated diffusion* and *active transport.*
5 Define and differentiate between *primary* and *secondary active transport.*
6 List three primary active transport carriers.
7 Differentiate between sodium *cotransport* and *countertransport.*
8 Define *osmosis.*
9 Define and differentiate between *molar concentration* and *osmolar concentration.*
10 Describe the effect of water and solute concentration on the direction of water movement across a membrane that is only permeable to water.
11 Describe the effects of *penetrating* and *nonpenetrating solutes* on cell volume.

12 Define *osmotic pressure, isotonic, hypotonic,* and *hypertonic solutions* and describe their effects on cell volume.

READING ASSIGNMENT

Chap. 6, pp. 120–134.

EXERCISES

PART I

Directions: Defend or refute the following statements.

1 Mediated transport is nothing more than simple diffusion of big molecules. **120**

2 The process of active transport wastes energy on the movement of molecules that would have moved by diffusion anyway. **123–125**

3 Osmosis is more like the simple diffusion of water then the active transport of water. **130**

4 Movement of molecules against their concentration gradient can only occur when mediated-transport mechanisms are present. **122–125**

5 Placing a red blood cell into pure water will cause the cell to lyse (burst), but placing a red blood cell into a 0.3 osmol solution of penetrating solute will cause the cell to shrink. **134**

PART II

130 Directions: Fill in the following table.

The Major Characteristics of Pathways by Which Substances Cross Membranes

	Diffusion			Mediated Transport	
	Through Lipid Bilayer	Through Protein Channel	Facilitated Diffusion	Primary Active Transport	Secondary Active Transport
Direction of net flux	______	High to low concentration	______	______	Low to high concentration
Equilibrium or steady state	$C_o = C_i$	______	______	$C_o \neq C_i$	______
Use of integral membrane protein	No	______	Yes	______	______
Saturation	______	No	______	Yes	______
Specificity	No	______	______	______	Yes
Use of energy source	______	No	No	______	______
Typical molecules using pathway	______ ______ ______	Ions: Na^+, K^+, Ca^{2+}	______ ______ ______	Ions: Na^+, Ca^{2+}, K^+	______ ______ ______

PART III

Directions: Complete the following items in the space provided.

1 Mediated-transport systems are distinguished from simple diffusion systems by having the characteristics of (a) ______________________ and (b)

121 ______________________.

2 When the maximum flux into or out of a cell is reached, the system is said to be

122 ______________________.

3 ________________ system is the class of mediated-transport systems that leads to equal concentrations of solute across the membrane. **122**

4 The reaction of solute with carrier must be asymmetric in ________________ systems. **123–124**

5 Primary active transport involves the ________________ use of ATP. **125**

6 ________________ involves the use of the concentration gradient for sodium (or some other ion) to supply energy for movement across the membrane. **125**

7 Secondary active transport can either be ________________ or ________________ depending on the relation to the sodium concentration gradient. **128–129**

8 During osmosis, water always moves from a region of ________________ solute concentration to a region of ________________ solute concentration. **130–134**

9 Extracellular fluid is a ________________ solution. **134**

SELF-TEST

PART I

Directions: Circle T for true and F for false.

T F 1 Large polar molecules require mediated-transport systems to enter cells.

T F 2 When a mediated-transport system is saturated, the flux is no longer proportional to the concentration gradient.

T F 3 Simple diffusion does not involve saturation or specificity.

T F 4 Phospholipids form the binding sites for mediated transport.

T F 5 Facilitated diffusion and active transport both move molecules "uphill" against concentration gradients.

T F 6 The affinity of the carrier for the solute must be different on the two sides of a membrane involved in active transport.

T F 7 Energy is only used in primary active transport not secondary active transport.

T F 8 Both primary and secondary active transport move solute against its concentration gradient.

T F 9 The movement of sodium is in opposite directions during cotransport and countertransport.

T F 10 When a cell is in osmotic equilibrium, the concentration of each solute is the same on both sides of the membrane.

T F 11 Only nonpenetrating or effectively nonpenetrating solutes can alter cell volume.

T F 12 For a given amount of glucose in solution the molar and osmolar concentrations are the same.

PART II

Directions: Circle the correct answer(s).

1 The following processes require the direct expenditure of metabolic energy:
   a osmosis
   b facilitated diffusion
   c active transport
   d simple diffusion
   e random movement of particles

2 Protein binding sites are responsible for
   a energy needed in transport process.
   b saturation of the mediated-transport system.
   c specificity of the mediated-transport system.
   d asymmetry in carrier affinity in active-transport systems.
   e regulation of membrane permeability characteristics.

Module III • Endocytosis, exocytosis, membrane junctions, epithelial transport, and glands

OBJECTIVES

Upon completion of this module, the student will be able to:

1 Define *endocytosis* and *exocytosis.*
2 Differentiate between *fluid* and *adsorptive endocytosis.*
3 Define and differentiate between *pinocytosis* and *phagocytosis.*
4 Describe the possible fates of material in an *endocytotic vesicle.*
5 Identify the two functions performed by exocytosis.
6 Describe the role of the *endoplasmic reticulum* and *Golgi apparatus* in protein secretion and membrane formation.
7 Describe the role of calcium in binding cells together.
8 Describe and differentiate among *desmosomes, tight junctions,* and *gap junctions.*
9 Differentiate between the *luminal* and *blood side* of epithelium.
10 Describe *epithelial transport* in terms of diffusion and mediated-transport systems.
11 Differentiate between *exocrine* and *endocrine glands.*

12 List the two categories of substances secreted by glands.
13 Differentiate between *apocrine secretions* and *holocrine secretions.*

READING ASSIGNMENT

Chap. 6, pp. 134–144.

EXERCISES

PART I

Directions: Defend or refute the following:

1 Exocytosis is nothing more than the cellular process of waste product disposal. **136–139**

____

____

____

2 Only the plasma membrane involved in endocytosis can be subsequently used for exocytosis.

____

____

____

3 The plasma membrane is the only membrane important to exocytotic and endocytotic activity.

____

____

____

PART II

Directions: Complete the following items in the space provided.

1 In the process of ____________________ the contents of the vesicle are the same as the contents of the extracellular fluid. **135**

2 A substance can be concentrated within the cell by the process of ____________________. **135**

3 The membrane that is removed from the cell surface by endocytosis is replaced by the process of ____________________. **136**

4 A vesicle containing a phagocytized bacterium would fuse with a(n) ______________________________, which would expose the bacterium to digestive enzymes.

5 The secretory function played by exocytosis is primarily involved in the secretion of ______________________________.

6 A(n) ______________________________ is a membrane junction characterized by a dense accumulation of matter between the membranes, which are separated by approximately 20 nm.

7 A membrane junction that involves an actual fusion of the outer protein surface of an adjacent membrane is a(n) ______________________________.

8 ______________________________ gland secretions flow through ducts.

9 ______________________________ secretion involves the complete disintegration of the cell.

PART III

Directions: Match the phrases in column B with the words in column A by writing the correct letter in the blank.

Column A		
1 ______	gap junction	**140**
2 ______	adsorptive endocytosis	**135**
3 ______	tight junctions	**139**
4 ______	lysosome	**135**
5 ______	pinocytosis protein	**135**
6 ______	phagocytosis	**135**
7 ______	desmosomes	**139**
8 ______	Golgi apparatus	**138**
9 ______	secretory granules	**137**
10 ______	calcium ions	**136**

Column B

a no space between cells
b cell drinking
c mechanical junctions
d allows transmission of electrical activity between cells
e progressively concentrates
f essential coupler in exocytosis
g protein-containing vesicles
h cell eating
i does the sorting and labeling of vesicles
j contain digestive enzymes

SELF-TEST

Directions: Circle T for true and F for false.

T F 1 A substance dissolves in the membrane as it is passed by endocytosis from the extracellular space to the intracellular space.

T F 2 Only vesicles formed by endocytosis can be released by exocytosis.

T F 3 Both endocytosis and exocytosis are examples of diffusion and, as such, require no metabolic energy source.

T F 4 Exocytosis can release both waste products and newly synthesized molecules.

T F 5 New cell surface membrane is formed by the endoplasmic reticulum and delivered to the surface during exocytosis.

T F 6 Tight junctions stop the movement of most large molecules between epithelial cells.

T F 7 The cytoplasms of adjacent cells are linked through gap junctions.

T F 8 Tight junctions permit the passage of electrical activity between adjacent cells.

T F 9 All endocytotic vesicles initially contain the same concentration of material as the extracellular fluid.

T F 10 The endoplasmic reticulum is formed by the remains of the plasma membranes that have undergone endocytosis.

T F 11 Exocrine glands secrete only by exocytosis.

T F 12 Apocrine secretion involves the complete disintegration of the cell.

T F 13 Endocrine glands function by endocytosis.

ANSWERS

CHAPTER 6 • MODULE I

PART I

1 F	(110)
2 F	(120)
3 F	(110)
4 F	(116)
5 T	(119)
6 F	(112)
7 T	(113)
8 T	(116)
9 T	(120)
10 F	(120)

PART II

1 b, d	(116)
2 a, b, c, d, e	(116–120)

CHAPTER 6 • MODULE II

PART I

1 T	(120–121)
2 T	(121–123)
3 T	(123)
4 F	(121)
5 F	(122–123)
6 T	(124)
7 F	(125)
8 T	(125)
9 F	(129)
10 F	(133)
11 T	(134)
12 T	(131)

PART II

1 c	(130)
2 b, c, d, e	(120–124)

CHAPTER 6 • MODULE III

1 F	(135)
2 F	(135–137)
3 F	(135–137)
4 T	(136–137)
5 T	(137–138)
6 T	(139)
7 T	(140)
8 F	(140)
9 F	(135)
10 F	(137–138)
11 F	(144)
12 F	(144)
13 F	(143–144)

7

HOMEOSTATIC MECHANISMS

Module I • General characteristics of homeostatic control systems
Module II • Balance concept and homeostatic systems
Module III • Receptors and postreceptor events

Module I • General characteristics of homeostatic control systems

OBJECTIVES

Upon completion of this module, the student will be able to:

1 Define *homeostasis.*
2 Describe the function of a *homeostatic mechanism.*
3 Define and describe the relation between *steady state* and the *operating point.*
4 Differentiate between *positive feedback* and *negative feedback.*
5 Define *error-signal* and state its role in feedback control.
6 Summarize the four generalizations about homeostatic control systems listed in Table 7-1, p. 148.
7 Define *acclimatization.*
8 Differentiate between *reversible* and *developmental acclimatizations.*
8 Define *biological rhythm.*
9 Describe the general characteristics of *aging.*

READING ASSIGNMENT

Chap. 7, pp. 147–153.

EXERCISES

PART I

Directions: Answer the following questions in the space provided.

1 Describe why perfect homeostasis is an ideal that can never be obtained. **150**

____

____

____

2 Describe the differences between the homeostatic mechanisms involved in temperature regulation and the acclimatization to an increase in environmental temperature. **151**

____

____

____

3 Describe why some forms of acclimatization are not reversible. **151**

____

____

____

4 Why do you think most biological control system have negative-feedback rather than positive-feedback components? **149–150**

____

____

____

PART II

Directions: Complete the following items in the space provided.

1 A ______________________ is a control system consisting of a collection of interconnecting components that function to keep a physical or chemical parameter of the body relatively constant. **147**

2 When a system is changing about its operating point such that input equals output, the system is said to be in ______________________. **148**

3 The major characteristic of a negative-feedback system is that it tends to push a variable (towards, away from) ______________________ the operating point rather than eliminate completely any change from the operating point. **148**

4 When an initial disturbance leads to a further increase in the disturbance, the system is said to be in ______________________________ feedback.

5 A change in an individual's ability to adapt to a particular environmental stress without a change in genetic endowment is called ______________________________.

6 The progressive failure of various homeostatic adaptive responses is the natural process of ______________________________.

SELF-TEST

PART I

Directions: Circle T for true and F for false.

T F 1 In a negative-feedback system the variable is prevented from changing from the operating point.

T F 2 In a homeostatic control system the receptor can be sensitive to variables outside or inside the body.

T F 3 Homeostatic control systems maintain the internal environment relatively constant.

T F 4 Only voluntary adjustments can occur in a homeostatic control system.

T F 5 The error-signal represents a biological defect in a homeostatic control system.

T F 6 Acclimatization is defined as an inherited biological adaptation to an environmental stress.

T F 7 Aging is a normal process that is generally not affected by environment.

PART II

Directions: Complete the following statements in the space provided.

1 The stability of a variable in the internal environment is achieved by balancing ______________________________ and ______________________________.

2 ______________________________ feedback displaces the system away from its steady-state operating point.

3 ______________________________ is a normal process that involves the gradual loss of the total number of cells in the body.

4 ______________________________ acclimatizations tend to be irreversible.

5 The difference between the operating point and the existing value of a biological variable is called the ______________________________.

Module II • Balance concept and homeostatic systems

OBJECTIVES

Upon completion of this module, the student will be able to:

1 Define *pool, net gain, net loss,* and *distribution* in the framework of *chemical homeostasis.*
2 Describe and diagram (according to Fig. 7-2, p. 154) the *balance concept.*
3 Distinguish between *total body balance* and *pool concentration.*
4 List *negative balance, positive balance,* and *balance* as the three possible states that can occur in total body balance and indicate how each state comes about.
5 Describe the two criteria necessary for a substance to be considered an *essential nutrient.*
6 Give the strict definition of a *reflex.*
7 Describe the characteristics of a *reflex response* that distinguish it from a *learned response.*
8 Define *stimulus, receptor, integrating center,* and *afferent and efferent pathway.*
9 Diagram the relationship among each of the five basic components of a *reflex arc.*
10 Compare the role of nerves and hormones in homeostatic control systems.
11 Describe a local homeostatic response and distinguish it from a reflex response.
12 Define *neurotransmitters, paracrines, autocrines,* and *nonspecific local messengers* and contrast their functions in homeostatic control systems.
13 Define *prostaglandins* and state the reason for their general importance in homeostatic control systems.
14 Identify the relationship between *arachidonic acid, cyclic endoperoxides, leukotrienes,* and *prostaglandins.*

READING ASSIGNMENT

Chap. 7, pp. 153–162.

EXERCISES

PART I

Directions: Answer the following questions in the space provided.

1 Describe why it is possible for the same individual to be in negative balance for one chemical and positive balance for another. 153–154

____

____

____

154–155 2 Explain why every complex molecule in our body is *not* an essential nutrient.

____

____

____

156 3 Draw and label the general components of a reflex arc.

161 4 Diagram the pathway for the synthesis of prostaglandins.

PART II

Directions: Complete the following items in the space provided.

1 The ______________________ is the body's readily available quan-
153 tity of a particular substance.

2 A chemical can be retained within the body but lost from the pool by being taken up in ______________________ or transformed into other ______
153–154 ______________.

3 Chemical homeostasis occurs in the presence of varying amounts of both input
154 and ______________________ from the pool.

4 An essential nutrient must be necessary for good health and inadequately ______
154 ______________________ by the body.

5 A system is in stable balance when ______________________ equals
154 ______________________.

6 When loss exceeds gain and the amount of the substance in the body is decreasing,
154 the system is said to be in ______________________.

7 The ______________________ is the pathway mediating a reflex re-
156 sponse.

8 ______________________ are specific chemical substances synthesized and secreted for the purpose of regulating local cells. **159**

9 Arachdonic acid is released from plasma membranes and is a precursor of ______ ______________ and ______________, which ultimately form all the members of the prostaglandin family. **161**

SELF-TEST

PART I

Directions: Circle T for true and F for false.

T F 1 Chemical homeostasis is responsible for maintaining some chemicals at absolutely constant concentrations in the body.

T F 2 During daily changes in body composition a homeostatic system can shift from positive to negative balance.

T F 3 The balance concept can be applied to both the physical variables and the amount of a chemical in the body.

T F 4 All the chemicals used in protein synthesis are essential nutrients.

T F 5 All essential nutrients are either proteins, carbohydrates, or fats

T F 6 Homeostatic control systems can alter balance by changing either gain or loss.

T F 7 Negative balance of an essential nutrient will ultimately lead to death.

T F 8 A stable balance can be disrupted by changes that occur external to the control system.

T F 9 The afferent and/or the efferent limb of a reflex can be operated by hormones rather than nerves.

T F 10 The pool readily receives from and contributes to all the other pathways involved in the balance schema.

T F 11 Most reflex responses must be learned.

T F 12 In a local response the entire sequence of events occurs within the area of the stimulus.

T F 13 The local release of hydrogen ions during metabolism is considered a paracrine function.

T F 14 Prostaglandins have been identified as having a primarily hormone-like function.

PART II

Directions: Answer the following questions in the space provided.

1 List the components of the reflex arc.

____

____

____

2 List the three possible states of total body balance.

____

____

____

PART III

Directions: Match the phrases in column B with the words in Column A by placing the correct letter on the line.

Column A	Column B
1 _______ reflex	a last component of a reflex arc
2 _______ effector	b minimizes change of a variable
3 _______ local response	c neither hormones nor nerves involved
4 _______ positive feedback	d receives multiple input from afferent pathways
5 _______ negative feedback	e normally activated by change of a variable
6 _______ integrator	f involuntary, unpremediated, unlearned
7 _______ receptor	g the value of a variable about which a control system operates
8 _______ stimulus	h leads to instability
9 _______ operating point	i a detectable change in the environment

Module III • Receptors and postreceptor events

OBJECTIVES

Upon completion of this module, the student will be able to:

1 Define *receptor*.
2 Describe the function and location of receptors and their role in determining the *specificity* of intercellular communication.
3 Describe *saturability* and *competition* in messenger-receptor interactions.
4 Define and differentiate between *agonists* and *antagonists* of chemical messengers.
5 Define and differentiate between *down-regulation* and *up-regulation* of receptors.
6 Define *supersensitivity*.

7 State the first step that is common to all messenger-receptor binding to plasma membranes.
8 List the two best understood sequences of postreceptor events initiated by binding of intercellular messengers to plasma membrane receptors.
9 Describe *receptor-operated channels.*
10 Describe the "*second messenger*" concept as it applies to cAMP and calcium and distinguish between first and second messengers.
11 List the sequence of events in the *cAMP* "second messenger" system.
12 Describe the role of activated *protein kinases* in the *amplification* of product molecule generation.
13 List the sequence of events in the *calcium* "second messenger" system.
14 Describe the role of *calcium-activated calmodulin* in cellular processes.
15 Describe the role of calcium as an *excitation-contraction coupler* and as an *excitation-secretion coupler.*
16 Describe the interaction of calcium and cAMP as second messengers.

READING ASSIGNMENT

Chap. 7, pp. 162–171.

EXERCISES

PART I

Directions: Answer the following questions in the space provided.

1 Describe the role of cAMP and protein kinases in intercellular communication. **165–166**

____

____

____

2 Defend or refute the position that the specificity of a cell's response is determined solely by the specificity of the plasma membrane receptor site. **162–167**

____

____

____

3 Describe two types of physiological regulation of receptors. **163**

____

____

____

163 4 Explain how down-regulation could be involved in disease.

____

____

____

5 Diagram the pathway by which calcium, via calmodulin, couples membrane events
169 to the cell's ultimate response.

PART II

Directions: Complete the following items in the space provided.

1 The three general types of intercellular transmitters are ________________
__________, ____________________, and ________________
162 ____________.

2 The receptors for intercellular transmitters can be located on the cell's ________
____________________ or in the ________________________ of
164 the cell.

3 The characteristic of a messenger-receptor interaction that allows certain cells
162 and not others to be influenced is called ____________________________.

4 A(n) ______________________________ is used to interfere with the action of
162–163 a particular messenger.

5 Cells exposed chronically to very low levels of a messenger may develop ______
163 __________________________ of the receptor for that messenger.

6 Calcium and cAMP are the two most widely studied _______________________
164 ______.

7 Activated adenylate cyclase catalyzes the conversion of ____________________
165 ____________ to __________________________________.

8 As a second messenger, calcium binds to ________________________________,
167 which in turn activates (or inhibits) ______________________________.

SELF-TEST

PART I

Directions: Circle T for true and F for false.

T F 1 Specificity is a characteristic that is imparted to a system only by the messenger.

T F 2 An agonist triggers a cell's response in exactly the same way as the true messenger.

T F 3 Down-regulation has the effect of reducing the target cell's response to a given messenger.

T F 4 All messengers bind to plasma membrane receptor sites.

T F 5 Phospholipid binding sites are the receptors for receptor-operated channels.

T F 6 The binding of messengers to certain plasma membrane receptors activates adenylate cyclase.

T F 7 The calcium and cAMP second messenger systems can only operate as totally independent systems.

T F 8 Receptor-operated channels can only change the movement of calcium through the membrane.

T F 9 The activation of protein kinase by cAMP is probably an event common to the biochemical sequences initiated by all cAMP-generating messengers.

T F 10 In chemical mediation the specificity of the response is a function of the second messenger.

T F 11 The same second messenger can initiate widely differing responses in different cells.

PART II

Directions: Fill in the missing steps in Fig. W-5.

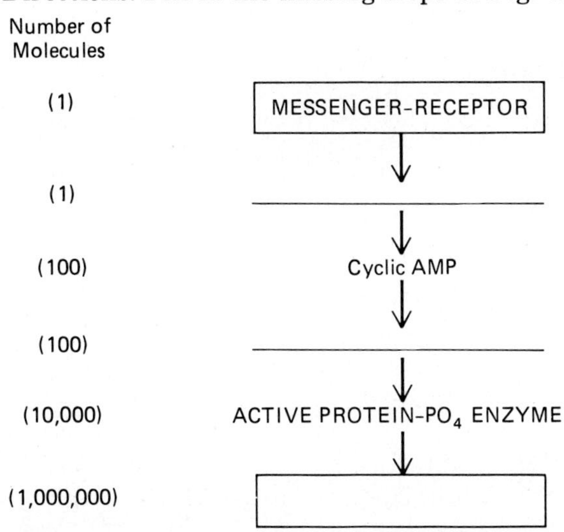

Fig. W-5: Amplification in the cAMP system.

Answers

CHAPTER 7 • MODULE I

PART I

1 F (150)
2 T (148)
3 T (150)
4 F (148)
5 F (150)
6 F (151)
7 F (152)

PART II

1 inputs, outputs (148)
2 positive (150)
3 aging (152)
4 developmental (151)
5 error/signal (150)

CHAPTER 7 • MODULE II

PART I

1 F (153)
2 T (154)
3 T (153–154)
4 F (154–155)
5 F (155)
6 T (154)
7 T (155)
8 T (155)
9 T (157)
10 T (154)
11 F (156)
12 T (159)
13 F (160)
14 F (162)

PART II

1 Receptor
Afferent pathway

PART III

1 f (156)
2 a (156)
3 c (159)
4 h (150)
5 b (148)
6 d (156)
7 e (156)
8 i (156)
9 g (148)

Integrating center
Efferent pathway
Effector (157)
2 Negative balance
Positive balance
Balance (154)

CHAPTER 7 • MODULE III

PART I

1 F (162)
2 T (163)
3 T (163)
4 F (164)
5 F (165)
6 T (165)
7 F (167–170)
8 F (165)
9 T (165–166)
10 F (162)
11 T (165–166)

PART II

See Fig. 7-12, p. 167

8
NEURAL CONTROL MECHANISMS

Module I • Structure of the nervous system
Module II • Electric potentials in the resting cell
Module III • Electric signals in the activated cell
Module IV • Synapses
Module V • Receptor activation and the flexion reflex

Module I • Structure of the nervous system

OBJECTIVES

Upon completion of this module, the student will be able to:

1 Define *neuron.*
2 List the four basic parts of the neuron.
3 Draw and label a nerve cell, including the *dendrites, cell body, initial segment, axon, axon collaterals*, and *axon terminals.*
4 Define *varicosities* and differentiate them from the axon terminal.
5 Distinguish between *projection neurons* and *local circuit neurons.*
6 Describe the structure and function of *myelin* and the *nodes of Ranvier.*
7 Define *axon transport.*
8 Describe the location and function of *afferent neurons, efferent neurons*, and *interneurons.*
9 Define *receptor, synapse, neurotransmitter, presynaptic neuron*, and *postsynaptic neuron.*
10 Differentiate between neurons and *glial cells* or *neuroglia* in terms of numbers, volume, and function in the nervous system.
11 Differentiate between the *central nervous system* and the *peripheral nervous system.*

12 Describe the basic functional anatomy of the *spinal cord* including the *gray matter, nuclei, white matter, tracts*, and *pathways*.
13 Describe the basic functional anatomy of *dorsal roots, dorsal root ganglia, ventral roots*, and *spinal nerves*.
14 List the six subdivisions of the brain.
15 List the components of the *brainstem* and the *forebrain*.
16 Differentiate among the *brainstem, cerebellum*, and *forebrain* by describing their general location and function.
17 Describe the location and general function of the *reticular formation*.
18 Identify the *commissures* and the *corpus callosum* as axon bundles that connect the right and left *cerebral hemispheres*.
19 Identify *association fibers* as axon bundles that connect areas within each of the hemispheres.
20 Define *cerebral cortex, thalamus, hypothalamus*, and *limbic system*.
21 Identify the components of the peripheral nervous system as the 31 pairs of *spinal nerves* and the 12 pairs of *cranial nerves*.
22 Describe the anatomy and function of neurons in the *afferent division* of the peripheral nervous system.
23 Differentiate between the *autonomic* and *somatic* subdivisions of the *efferent division* of the peripheral nervous system.
24 Define *motor neuron* and identify its function and neurotransmitter.
25 Compare the *preganglionic* and *postganglionic* cell body location and neurotransmitters released in the *sympathetic* and *parasympathetic* divisions of the autonomic nervous systems.
26 Define *adrenergic* and *cholinergic* fibers.
27 Differentiate between *nicotinic receptors* and *muscarinic receptors*.
28 Differentiate between *alpha-adrenergic receptors* and *beta-adrenergic receptors*.
29 Describe the relationship between the *adrenal medulla* and the sympathetic nervous system.
30 Define and give examples of *dual innervation*.
31 List the effects of the sympathetic and parasympathetic nervous systems as outlined in Table 8-4, pp. 188–189.
32 Describe the function of the *blood–brain barrier*.
33 Describe the movement of *cerebrospinal fluid* from the *choroid plexuses* through the *cerebral ventricles* and ultimately back into the large veins on the surface of the brain.

READING ASSIGNMENT

Chap. 8, pp. 172–190.

EXERCISES

Directions: Answer the following questions in the space provided.

1 Draw and label a "typical" neuron. **Fig. 8-1, p. 174**

What specializations would you expect in each of the elements depicted in your drawing

a if the neuron were an afferent neuron?

____

____

____

b if the neuron were an efferent neuron?

____

____

____

c if the neuron were an interneuron?

____

____

______________________________ **174–177**

2 List the six major subdivisions of the central nervous system. **178**

____

____

____

3 List the divisions of the peripheral nervous system. **Table 8-2, 183**

____

____

____

4 List three distinguishing characteristics of the:
a somatic nervous system

____

____

____

Table 8-3, p. 184 b autonomic nervous system

____

____

____

5 List the two general types of adrenergic receptors.

a _______________

185 b _______________

6 List the two general types of cholinergic receptors.

a _______________

184–185 b _______________

7 Complete the following outline of the major division of the nervous system. Then
174–184 answer the following questions in the spaces provided.

I Central nervous system (CNS)

II

A Afferent

B

1

2

a

b sympathetic

a Which of the above groups conveys information from receptors to the central nervous system?

____

Where are its cell bodies located?

____

b Which group leaves the CNS to innervate skeletal muscle?

____

How many neurons are in this pathway?

____

c Which of the autonomic fibers are also known as the thoracolumbar division?

____

Where do their cell bodies lie in relation to the spinal cord?

____

This system functions in what type of situation?

____

Give an example.

____

8 What is the significance of dual innervation in the autonomic nervous system? **186**

____

____

____

SELF-TEST

PART I

Directions: Circle T for true and F for false.

T F 1 The number of neurons is approximately equal to the number of glia in the nervous system.
T F 2 Most axons and dendrites are approximately the same length.
T F 3 Most neurons function as both afferent and efferent neurons.
T F 4 Organs that are innervated by both the sympathetic and parasympathetic systems are said to receive dual innervation.
T F 5 Somatic efferent neurons synapse just outside the spinal cord prior to reaching the effector organs.
T F 6 The transmitter released from the parasympathetic fibers at the effector organ is acetylcholine.
T F 7 Afferent information enters the spinal cord through the dorsal roots.
T F 8 Parasympathetic effects on the heart are a decreased heart rate and increased contractility.

PART II

Directions: Complete the following items in the space provided.

1 Another name for the parasympathetic division of the autonomic nervous system is the _______________ division.

2 Most ascending and descending tracts are located in the _______________ of the spinal cord.

3 Many harmful substances are prevented from reaching neural tissue of the brain by the _______________ barrier.

4 The ventricles of the brain are perfused by ______________________ fluid.

5 The reticular formation is located in the ______________________.

PART III

Directions: Circle the correct answer(s).

1 Which of the following responses is (are) initiated by parasympathetic stimulation?
   a dilation of the pupils
   b increased stomach motility
   c constriction of arterioles in the skin
   d stimulation of insulin secretion
2 Which of the following responses is (are) initiated by sympathetic stimulation?
   a secretion by the adrenal medulla
   b decreased contractility of the heart
   c relaxation of the bladder sphincter
   d increased heart rate
3 An important integrating center for most sensory input on its way to the cortex is the
   a basal ganglia. b cerebellum. c thalamus. d hypothalamus.
4 Which of the following has its chief role in maintaining balance and coordination of muscle movement?
   a reticular formation b cerebellum c thalamus d cerebrum

Module II • Electric potentials in the resting cell

OBJECTIVES

Upon completion of this module, the student will be able to:

1 Define *electric potential, potential difference, resistance,* and *current* and state their relationship as given by *Ohm's law.*
2 Differentiate between an *insulating* material and a *conducting* material and give examples of each in a biological system.
3 Describe the *resting cell membrane potential* by giving the orientation and magnitude of the potential as well as the two points across which it is measured.
4 Define the *diffusion potential.*
5 Describe the effect of membrane permeability and concentration gradients on the diffusion potential.

6 Define *equilibrium potential.*
7 Differentiate between concentration force and electric force as each contributes to the equilibrium potential.
8 Describe the resting membrane potential and the potassium equilibrium potential, and give the reason why they are not the same.
9 Define *electrogenic pump.*
10 Describe the role of the *Na,K-pump* in contributing to the resting membrane potential.
11 Identify the relationship between the chloride equilibrium potential and the resting membrane potential.

READING ASSIGNMENT

Chap. 8, pp. 190–196.

EXERCISES

PART I

Directions: Answer the following questions in the space provided.

1 Write Ohm's law and define each term. **191**

____

____

____

2 Describe the factors that determine the equilibrium potential for any given ion. **193**

____

____

____

3 What would happen to the resting membrane potential if the cell membrane were more permeable to sodium than to potassium? Why? **192–193**

____

____

____

PART II

Directions: Complete the following items in the space provided.

1 The resting membrane potential is closer to the ______________________________ equilibrium potential than to the ______________________________ equilibrium potential. **195**

2 Even with a stable resting membrane potential some potassium is leaking
________________ the cell, and some sodium is leaking
195 ________________ the cell.

3 The "leaks" in the membrane do not destroy the cell because normal concentra-
195–196 tion gradients are maintained by ________________.

4 The resting membrane is more permeable to ________________
195 than to ________________.

5 At the equilibrium potential the concentration forces are balanced by the
193 ________________ forces acting across the membrane.

SELF-TEST

Directions: Circle T for true and F for false.

T F 1 If the potassium permeability alone were to increase, the membrane potential would become more negative.

T F 2 Destruction of the membrane pump results in the immediate reduction of the membrane potential to zero.

T F 3 The membrane potential must be at either the potassium equilibrium potential or the sodium equilibrium potential.

T F 4 If a membrane were at the potassium equilibrium potential, there would be no net diffusion of potassium.

T F 5 Membrane pumps contribute indirectly to the membrane potential by maintaining the concentration gradients across the membrane.

T F 6 Increasing the permeability of the membrane to ions decreases the insulating function of the membrane.

Module III • Electric signals in the activated cell

OBJECTIVES

Upon completion of this module, the student will be able to:

1 Define the changes in membrane potential when the membrane is said to be *depolarized, hyperpolarized*, and *repolarized.*
2 Define *graded potential* and state the relationship between the amplitude of this potential and the events that initiate the change.

3 Define *decremental conduction* and state the consequences of such conduction to signal transmission.
4 Define *excitable membrane.*
5 Describe the magnitude and direction of the changes in sodium and potassium permeability during the rising phase, the falling phase, and the *after hyperpolarization* of the *action potential.*
6 Describe and diagram the positive-feedback relationship in the rising phase of the action potential.
7 Describe *voltage-sensitive ion channels.*
8 Describe the relationship between the *threshold potential* and the occurrence of the action potential.
9 Distinguish between *suprathreshold* and *subthreshold stimuli* and between *threshold* and *subthreshold potentials.*
10 Describe the *all-or-none* nature of the action potential.
11 Define *refractory period.*
12 Distinguish between *relative* and *absolute refractory* periods.
13 Describe action-potential propagation and differentiate this process from decremental conduction by discussing the amplitude and direction of each.
14 Describe two factors affecting the velocity of action potentials.
15 Diagram and define *saltatory conduction.*
16 Define *pacemaker potential.*

READING ASSIGNMENT

Chap. 8, pp. 196–207.

EXERCISES

Directions: Answer the following questions in the space provided.

1 Draw a graph of a membrane potential of a nerve cell versus time in milliseconds, including the resting membrane potential, sodium equilibrium potential, and potassium equilibrium potential. Show graphically what happens to the membrane potential of this neuron when the cell is depolarized to the threshold potential and when the cell is hyperpolarized. **193–194, 200**

2 Defend the position: Although both graded potentials and action potentials are important in information processing, the action potential is essential to homeo-
196–199 stasis in a multiorgan animal.

____

____

____

3 Diagram the positive-feedback system that is activated during an action poten-
202 tial.

200 4 Fill in the table below comparing the graded potential with the action potential.

	Graded Potentials	Action Potentials
a	graded response	____________ response
b	can be summed	____________ be summed
c	____________	threshold 10–15 mV from resting membrane potential
d	____________ conduction	conducted with constant amplitude
e	____________	duration constant
f	depolarization or hyperpolerization	____________

5 Diagram the changes in membrane permeability to sodium and potassium that
201 occur with the membrane potential changes during the action potential.

SELF-TEST

PART I

Directions: Circle T for true and F for False.

T F 1 The critical level to which the membrane must be depolarized to trigger an action potential is known as the threshold potential.

T F 2 When the membrane is being depolarized, the potential is less negative than the resting membrane potential.

T F 3 All graded potentials result in action potentials.

T F 4 Decremental conduction transmits a depolarization over the entire length of an axon.

T F 5 The sodium permeability and potassium permeability change to about the same extent and at the same time during an action potential.

T F 6 The larger the receptor potential, the larger the action potential.

T F 7 The reversal in membrane potential that occurs during an action potential is caused by a reversal of the chemical concentration gradients.

T F 8 The after hyperpolarization results from an elevated potassium permeability.

T F 9 The absolute refractory period limits the number of action potentials that can occur in a given period of time.

T F 10 Larger diameter fibers generally transmit action potentials faster than do smaller diameter fibers.

PART II

Directions: Complete the following items in the space provided.

1 Nerve and muscle cells transmit electrical information by ______ potentials and by ______ potentials.

2 A stimulus to a nerve or muscle cell that does not reach threshold is termed ______.

3 In the initial stages of the action potential the permeability of the membrane to sodium increases ______-fold.

4 Stimuli that are more than the threshold magnitude are called ______.

5 Once a threshold level has been reached, the action potential that results is described as a(n) ______ response.

PART III

Directions: Circle the correct answer(s).

1 The speed at which an action potential is transmitted depends on
   a fiber diameter.
   b fiber length.
   c whether or not the fiber is myelinated.
   d the number of branches along the membrane.

2 The relative refractory period corresponds to
   a decreased potassium permeability.
   b increased potassium permeability.
   c sodium permeability changes.
   d threshold potential that is further from zero.
   e threshold potential that is closer to zero.

3 A myelinated nerve is associated with
   a saltatory conduction.
   b decreased local current flow.
   c slower action-potential conduction.
4 Excitable membranes
   a are present on all membrane-bound tissues.
   b are responsible for the cell's ability to produce action potentials.
   c require myelin to act as an insulator for electrical events.
   d can experience a reversal of the electric potential across the membrane.
   e are generally impermeable to both Na and K ions.

Module IV • Synapses

OBJECTIVES

Upon completion of this module, the student will be able to:

1 Define *synapse.*
2 Differentiate between an *excitatory* and an *inhibitory synapse.*
3 Differentiate between *presynaptic neurons* and *postsynaptic neurons.*
4 Describe *convergence, divergence*, and *neural integration.*
5 Differentiate between *electric* and *chemical synapses.*
6 Diagram and describe a synapse including the concepts of *axon terminal, synaptic cleft, synaptic vesicles, subsynaptic membrane, one-way conduction*, and *synaptic delay.*
7 List the three mechanisms by which the transmitter is removed from the subsynaptic membrane.
8 Describe the changes in resting membrane potential of a postsynaptic cell at an excitatory synapse and at an inhibitory synapse.
9 Differentiate between *temporal summation* and *spatial summation* and describe their relationship to *facilitation, inhibition*, and *excitation* of the neuron.
10 Describe the functional significance of the lower threshold of the *initial segment.*
11 Describe the integrator function of a postsynaptic cell using the concepts in objectives 8, 9, and 10.
12 List three factors that affect the amount of neurotransmitter at a synapse.
13 Define *presynaptic inhibition* and *presynaptic facilitation.*
14 Differentiate presynaptic inhibition from an inhibitory postsynaptic potential.
15 List the four general classes of neurotransmitters and identify examples of each.
16 Discuss the synthesis and degradation of acetylcholine.
17 List the steps of catecholamine synthesis, storage, release, action, reuptake, and degradation.

18 List the 11 sites of drug action at the synapse (Fig. 8-46, p. 217).
19 Differentiate between *neurotransmitters* and neuromodulators.
20 Define *neuroeffector junction* and give two examples of neuroeffector transmitters.

READING ASSIGNMENT

Chap. 8, pp. 207–219.

EXERCISES

Directions: Answer the following questions in the space provided.

1 Draw and label a chemical synapse. What is the function of each component you have labeled? **208**

2 How do ESPSs and IPSPs differ? Why are both types of postsynaptic potentials necessary? **209–210**

3 Describe the importance of the initial segment of the neuron to the integrator function of the cell body. **211–212**

4 Define temporal and spatial summation by drawing the effects of multiple IPSPs and EPSPs on the resting membrane potential. **211–212**

5 Explain the differences among neurotransmitter, hormone, and neuromodulator. **218**

SELF-TEST

PART I

Directions: Match the items in Column B with those in Column A by inserting the most appropriate letter in the space provided.

Column A	Column B
1 ______ convergence	a contains receptor sites for released transmitter
2 ______ electric synapse	b depends primarily on the frequency of synaptic events
3 ______ subsynaptic membrane	c a subthreshold event
4 ______ temporal summation	d principal site of action-potential formation
5 ______ facilitation	e multiple synapses on a single cell
6 ______ initial segment	f synaptic mechanisms
7 ______ presynaptic inhibition	g stores neurotransmitter
8 ______ site of drug action	h local current flows directly through gap junctions
9 ______ synaptic vesicles	i hyperpolarization
10 ______ inhibitory postsynaptic potential	j modifies transmitter release

PART II

Directions: Circle the correct answer(s).

1 Which of the following are known or presumed to be neurotransmitters?
a serotonin b acetylcholine c norepinephrine d dopamine

2 A general depolarization of the membrane when excitatory synaptic activity predominates is known as
a temporal summation. b facilitation. c IPSP. d convergence.

3 Synaptic delay is primarily a result of the
a width of the synaptic cleft.
b permeability changes in the postsynaptic membrane.
c release mechanism that frees the transmitter.
d time necessary for transmitter diffusion.

4 Which of the following are involved in the integrator function of nerve cells?
a facilitation
b temporal summation
c spatial summation
d convergence
e divergence

PART III

Directions: Circle T for true and F for false.

T F 1 An EPSP results from an increase in the membrane's permeability to positively charged ions.
T F 2 Glycine is thought to be a neurotransmitter.
T F 3 An IPSP leads to a slight depolarization of the postsynaptic membrane.
T F 4 Synaptic events last the same length of time as an action potential.
T F 5 The effectiveness of a synaptic connection is fixed.

PART IV

Directions: Complete the following items in the space provided.

1 Membrane-enclosed structures that contain the transmitter are termed ______________________________.

2 Summation due to EPSPs at different places on the postsynaptic neuron is called ______________________________.

3 Chemicals released from efferent neurons to alter the activity of glands or muscle cells are known as ______________________________.

4 A synapse can conduct only in one direction because the ______________________________ are on one side and the ______________________________ are on the other.

5 A slight depolarization of the cell membrane that leads to a decrease in the amount of transmitter released at the synapse is termed ______________________________.

Module V • Receptor activation and the flexion reflex

OBJECTIVES

Upon completion of this module, the student will be able to:

1 Define *receptor* and describe its role in the process of *transduction* of energy.
2 Describe the *doctrine of specific nerve energies.*
3 Describe the formation and function of a *receptor potential.*
4 Describe how action-potential frequency is determined by the amplitude and duration of the receptor potential.
5 Describe how stimulus intensity and rate of stimulus application vary the amplitude of the receptor potential.

6 Describe how *summation* and *adaptation* alter the amplitude and duration of the receptor potential.
7 Define *sensory unit, stimulus modality*, and *receptive field.*
8 List the three basic characteristics of sensory coding.
9 Describe how coding of a stimulus intensity is accomplished by the *firing frequency* and *recruitment* of neurons.
10 Describe how different degrees of *stimulus localization* are produced.
11 Define *disinhibition* and *lateral inhibition.*
12 Describe the *flexion reflex* including a discussion of *polysynaptic reflexes, reciprocal innervation*, and *crossed-extensor reflex.*

READING ASSIGNMENT

Chap. 8, pp. 219–228.

EXERCISES

Directions: Answer the following questions in the space provided.

220–221 1 If a receptor potential does not always result in an action potential, is there not a waste of membrane activity?

____

____

____

222–225 2 Describe the difference between stimulus modality and stimulus localization.

____

____

____

207, 223–224 3 Describe the difference between recruitment and convergence.

____

____

____

228 4 Diagram the polysynaptic spinal reflex involved in withdrawing one's hand or foot from a sharp object.

SELF-TEST

PART I

Directions: Circle T for true and F for false.

T F 1 The amplitude and duration of the receptor potential will determine the frequency of action potentials.

T F 2 Action potentials generally do not originate within the receptor membrane because this region has a very high threshold.

T F 3 A single larger receptor potential can initiate several action potentials in that axon.

T F 4 Receptor potentials travel by decremental conduction.

T F 5 Some receptor potentials are decreased by adaptation.

T F 6 The amplitude of the receptor potential increases with a greater rate of stimulation.

T F 7 Receptor potentials may be summed resulting in a larger depolarization.

T F 8 Adaptation is a decrease in the frequency of action potentials in the afferent neuron despite a constant stimulus magnitude.

T F 9 Most receptors respond equally to all types of energy.

T F 10 One way of intensity coding in a single axon is accomplished by varying the action-potential frequency.

T F 11 Recruitment involves the activation of additional afferent neurons.

T F 12 Different types of stimuli result in different types of action potentials.

PART II

Directions: Fill in the correct answer in the space provided.

1 The coding of afferent information is accomplished by ____________________,

____________________, and ____________________.

2 The ____________________ of a sensory neuron is that area of the body that, if stimulated, leads to activity in the neuron.

3 The process by which stimulus energy is transformed into electrical responses is known as ____________________.

4 ____________________ enhances the stronger inputs, and the weaker inputs of adjacent sensory units are simultaneously inhibited.

5 The inhibition of antagonistic motor neurons is called ____________________.

Answers

CHAPTER 8 • MODULE I

PART I

1 F (176)
2 F (173)
3 F (174)
4 T (185)
5 F (183)
6 T (184)
7 T (177)
8 F (188)

PART II

1 craniosacral (184)
2 white matter (177)
3 blood–brain (189)
4 cerebrospinal (189)
5 brainstem (178)

PART III

1 b (188)
2 a, d (185, 188)
3 c (180)
4 b (179)

CHAPTER 8 • MODULE II

1 T (193)
2 F (195-196)
3 F (193)
4 T (193)
5 T (196)
6 T (191)

CHAPTER 8 • MODULE III

PART I

1 T (202)
2 T (196)
3 F (196–198)
4 F (199)
5 F (201)
6 F (203)
7 F (200–201)
8 T (201)
9 T (203)
10 T (206)

PART II

1 graded, action (196–199)
2 subthreshold (202–203)
3 several hundred (201)
4 suprathreshold stimuli (203)
5 all-or-none (203)

PART III

1 a, c (205–206)
2 b, e (203–204)
3 a, b (205–206)
4 b, d (199,205)

CHAPTER 8 • MODULE IV

PART I

1 e (207)
2 h (207)
3 a (209)
4 b (211)
5 c (211)
6 d (212)
7 j (213–214)
8 f (217)
9 g (208–209)
10 i (209–210)

PART II

1 a, b, c, d (214)
2 b (211)
3 c (209)
4 a, b, c, d, e (207, 210–212)

PART III

1 T (209)
2 T (214)
3 F (210)
4 F (209)
5 F (212–213)

PART IV

1 synaptic vesicles (208)
2 spatial summation (211)
3 neuroeffector transmitters (219)
4 synaptic vesicles; receptor sites (209)
5 presynaptic inhibition (214)

CHAPTER 8 • MODULE V

PART I

1 T (221)
2 T (221)
3 T (221)
4 T (221)
5 T (221)
6 T (221)
7 T (221)
8 T (221–222)
9 F (219)
10 T (223)
11 T (223–224)
12 F (223)

PART II

1 stimulus modality, stimulus intensity, stimulus localization (222)
2 receptive field (222)
3 transduction (219)
4 lateral inhibition (227)
5 reciprocal innervation (228)

9
HORMONAL CONTROL MECHANISMS

Module I • General principles of endocrinology
Module II • Control of hormone secretion

Module I • General principles of endocrinology

OBJECTIVES

Upon completion of this module, the student will be able to:

1 Define *hormone, endocrine, neurohormone,* and *neuroendocrinology.*
2 Given a list of endocrine glands, state (a) the hormones each gland secretes and (b) the major functions of each of these hormones.
3 State the significance of *hormone-target-cell specificity.*
4 For the following hormones, state whether they fall into the general classes of (a) amines, (b) peptides or proteins, or (c) steroids: thyroxine (T_4), triiodothyronine (T_3), calcitonin, aldosterone, cortisol, corticosterone, dehydroepiandrosterone, testosterone, and estrogen.
5 Describe the role of *prohormones* in the synthesis of peptide hormones.
6 Distinguish between a *mineralocorticoid* and a *glucocorticoid.*
7 Define *androgen.*
8 Define *effective* and *total plasma concentration* of a hormone.
9 List and describe the general factors that determine the plasma concentrations of hormones.
10 List the four general fates of hormones following secretion as depicted in Fig. 9-6, p. 238.

11 State that the end result of the action of a hormone is an alteration in the rate at which the target cells perform a specific function.
12 Describe the role of hormone receptors in hormone action.
13 List the cellular locations of the receptor site for most steroid hormones and for most nonsteroid hormones.
14 Compare the mechanism of action of steroid hormones with that of peptide hormones.
15 Describe the phenomenon of *permissiveness* and the *pharmacological* effects of hormones.

READING ASSIGNMENT

Chap. 9, pp. 229–240.

EXERCISES

PART I

Directions: Answer the following items in the space provided.

(232–233) 1 Fill in the blank spaces in the following table.

Gland	Hormone	Major Function Is Control of
____________	Releasing hormones	Secretion by the anterior pituitary
	Oxytocin	(See posterior pituitary)
	Vasopressin (antidiuretic hormone, ADH)	(See posterior pituitary)
Anterior pituitary	Growth hormone (somatotropin, GH, STH)	Growth; organic metabolism
	Thyroid-stimulating hormone (TSH, thyrotropin)	____________
	Adrenocorticotropic hormone (ACTH, corticotropin)	____________
	Prolactin	____________
	Gonadotropic hormones: Follicle-stimulating hormone (FSH) Luteinizing hormone (LH)	____________

Gland	Hormone	Major Function Is Control of
Posterior pituitary	________	Milk "let-down;" uterine motility
	________	Water excretion
Adrenal cortex	________	Organic metabolism; response to stress
	________	Growth and, in women, sexual activity
	________	Sodium and potassium excretion
Adrenal medulla	________	Organic metabolism; cardiovascular function; response to stress
	________	
Thyroid	________	Energy metabolism; growth
	________	
	________	Plasma calcium
________	Parathyroid hormone (parathormone, PTH, PH)	Plasma calcium and phosphate
Gonads		
Female: ovaries	________	Reproductive system; growth and development breasts
Male: testes	________	Reproductive system; growth and development
Pancreas	________	Organic metabolism; plasma glucose
	________	
	________	
Kidney	________	Adrenal cortex, blood pressure
	Erythropoietin	________
	1,25-Dihydroxyvitamin D_3	________
Gastrointestinal tract	Gastrin	________
	Secretin	
	Cholecystokinin	
	Gastric inhibitory peptide	
	Somatostatin	
Liver	Somatomedin	________

Gland	Hormone	Major Function Is Control of
Thymus	Thymus hormone (thymosin)	____________
Pineal	____________	Sexual maturity
Placenta	Chorionic gonadotropin Estrogens, Progesterone	____________

237 2 Describe why the effective plasma concentration of steroid hormones is often less than the total plasma concentration of that hormone.

____

____

____

233–235 3 For each of the following hormones state whether they fall into the category of amines, peptides or proteins, or steroids.

a thyroid hormone

____

b epinephrine

____

c aldosterone

____

d calcitonin

____

e cortisol

____

237–238 4 Describe the general factors that determine the plasma concentration of hormones.

____

____

____

238–239 5 Describe how changes in receptors can affect hormonal action.

____

____

____

6 Describe what is meant by the pharmacological effect of hormones. **240**

____

____

____

PART II

Directions: Define the following terms.

1 hormone ____________________

____________________ **229**

2 endocrine ____________________

____________________ **229**

3 neuroendocrinology ____________________

____________________ **230**

4 neurohormone ____________________

____________________ **229**

5 prohormone ____________________

____________________ **234**

6 permissiveness ____________________

____________________ **239–240**

SELF-TEST

PART I

Directions: complete the following items in the space provided.

1 Administration of a large quantity of a hormone may have results that are never seen in a normal person; these results are called ____________________ effects.

2 Hormones that must be present (usually in small quantities) to enable other hormones to exert their full effects exhibit the phenomenon known as ____________________.

3 A hormone is defined as a chemical substance synthesized by an ____________________

______________ gland and carried by the ______________ to other sites in the body where its actions are exerted.

4 The interrelationship between endocrine function and the brain is known as ______________.

5 The general factors that determine the blood concentration of hormones are ______________, ______________, and ______________.

6 The receptors for steroid hormones are located ______________.

7 The receptors for most protein hormones are located ______________.

8 A common denominator of the effects of the steroid hormones is an increased synthesis of ______________.

PART II

Directions: Circle the correct answer(s).

1 The following are hormones produced in the anterior pituitary:
  a parathyroid hormone
  b antidiuretic hormone
  c adrenocorticotropic hormone
  d renin
  e luteinizing hormone

2 Which of the following glands and functions are correct?
  a hypothalamic area that produces releasing hormones—control of secretion of the anterior pituitary
  b adrenal medulla—organic metabolism; cardiovascular function; response to stress
  c parathyroids—plasma calcium and phosphate regulation
  d thymus—lymphocyte development
  e pancreas—milk secretion

3 Which of the following are hormones secreted by the gastrointestinal tract?
  a insulin
  b androgens
  c cholecystokinin
  d somatostatin
  e gastrin

4 Which of the following hormones are secreted from the adrenal *cortex?*
  a cortisol
  b oxytocin
  c epinephrine
  d aldosterone
  e androgens

Module II • Control of hormone secretion

OBJECTIVES

Upon completion of this module, the student will be able to:

1 Describe why the concentration of a hormone often varies over a brief time span.
2 Describe and give examples of the four general types of direct control of endocrine cells that can result in changes in hormonal secretion.
3 State the importance of negative feedback in the regulation of hormone secretion.
4 Define *tropic* hormone.
5 Describe the general anatomy of the posterior and anterior pituitary glands.
6 List the two peptide hormones produced in the hypothalamus and stored in the posterior pituitary.
7 Describe how the hormones oxytocin and ADH move from the hypothalamus to the posterior pituitary.
8 State the type of input controlling the secretion of hormones from the posterior hypothalamus.
9 List the six classic hormones produced by the anterior pituitary gland and their major functions.
10 List two peptides cosecreted with ACTH.
11 Describe the role of the hypothalamus and the hypothalamo-pituitary portal vessels in the regulation of anterior pituitary hormone secretion.
12 List the hypothalamic releasing hormones (including the hypothalamic hormones, which inhibit the release of the anterior pituitary hormones) and describe their function.
13 Describe the neural and hormonal control of hypothalamic releasing hormones.
14 Contrast "long-loop" with "short-loop" negative feedback in the control of hormone secretion.
15 Describe the control systems involving ACTH, TSH, and GH.
16 Describe the major functions of cortisol.
17 Describe the hypothesized roles of β-endorphin.
18 Describe the various stages in the development of *iodine-deficiency goiter.*

READING ASSIGNMENT

Chap. 9, pp. 240–254.

EXERCISES

PART I

Directions: Answer the following questions in the space provided.

1 On the basis of your knowledge of negative feedback in the control of hormone secretion, predict the effects of the following on the rates of secretion of releasing factors, pituitary hormones, and target-gland hormones for the control system in-
248–253 volving ACTH, TSH, and GH:

a destroying the hypothalamic area responsible for producing the releasing factors

____

____

b destroying the anterior pituitary gland

____

____

c injecting purified anterior pituitary hormones into an individual

____

____

2 Using the concept of hormonal feedback, describe the pathway to the development
252 of iodine-deficiency goiter.

____

____

____

250 3 Describe the difference between long-loop and short-loop negative feedback.

____

____

____

4 Describe the possible reasons for a patient having an unusually low plasma con-
238, centration of cortisol.
448–250

____

____

____

252 5 A person is receiving large quantities of thyroid hormones.

a Will the individual's thyroid gland be producing smaller amounts of thyroid hormones (compared with preinjection levels)? Why?

____

b What will be the effect of these high plasma levels of thyroid hormones on the secretion rates of TSH?

____

SELF-TEST

PART I

Directions: Complete the following items in the space provided.

1 Name the system that provides for communicaton between the hypothalamus and the anterior pituitary. ______________________

2 Oxytocin and ADH are synthesized within the ______________________.

3 The secretion of epinephrine by the adrenal medulla is dependent on stimulation of ______________________.

4 The posterior pituitary is an outgrowth of the ______________________.

5 Specific inputs that affect secretion of a particular hormone include ______________________, ______________________, ______________________, ______________________, and ______________________.

6 The situation where a hormone secreted by a peripheral endocrine gland exerts negative feedback over the anterior pituitary or the hypothalamus is known as ______________________.

7 Hypothesized roles for β-endorphin include ______________________, ______________________, and ______________________.

PART II

Directions: Circle the correct answer(s).

1 Which of the following hormones are produced by the anterior pituitary?
a β-lipotrophin b growth hormone c insulin d ACTH e prolactin

2 The anterior pituitary gland
a receives hormonal input from the hypothalamus.
b receives neural input from the hypothalamus.
c stores oxytocin and ADH.
d produces releasing hormones.

3 Which of the following are tropic hormones?
a ACTH
b prolactin
c FSH
d TSH
e GH

4 If the feedback loop were broken between the hypothalamic area responsible for the secretion of the releasing hormones and the anterior pituitary gland (e.g., by some surgical procedure), which of the following would occur?
   a Blood levels of cortisol would go up.
   b Iodine-deficiency goiter would develop.
   c Blood concentration of ACTH would decrease.
   d Blood thyroid hormones concentration would rise.

5 Following the surgical removal of the anterior pituitary,
   a blood concentration of ACTH would rise.
   b the hypothalamo-anterior-pituitary portal vessel concentration of CRH would fall.
   c blood concentration of somatomedin would fall.
   d blood concentration of cortisol would fall.

Answers

CHAPTER 9 • MODULE I

PART I

1 pharmacological (240)
2 permissiveness (239–240)
3 endocrine; blood (229)
4 neurendocrinology (230)
5 rates of secretion, rates of inactivation, rates of excretion (237)
6 within the cell (239)
7 on the cell surface or plasma membrane (239)
8 proteins (239)

PART II

1 c, e (244–245)
2 a, b, c, d (232–233)
3 c, d, e (232)
4 a, d,e (232)

CHAPTER 9 • MODULE II

PART I

1 hypothalamo-pituitary portal vessels (246)
2 hypothalamus (243)
3 sympathetic nerves to the adrenal medulla (242)
4 hypothalamus (243)
5 changes in concentrations of mineral ions or organic nutrients, neural input, another hormone (in any order) (241)
6 long-loop negative feedback (250)
7 effects on pain perception, appetite, learning (in any order) (251)

PART II

1 b, d, e (246)
2 a (244–247)
3 a, c, d, e (243, 245–246)
4 c (249–253)
5 c, d (245–253)

10
MUSCLE

Module I • General structure and function of muscle
Module II • Excitation and contraction of muscle fibers
Module III • Muscle mechanics and metabolism
Module IV • Characteristics of differentiated muscles

Module I • General structure and function of muscle

OBJECTIVES

Upon completion of this module, the student will be able to:

1 State that muscle cells have *specialized* ability to generate force and motion.
2 List and describe the general location and function of the three types of muscle cells.
3 Differentiate between a *muscle fiber* and a *muscle.*
4 Describe *striated muscle* and the intracellular elements responsible for the striations.
5 Differentiate between *myofibrils* and *muscle filaments.*
6 Define *sarcomere* and list each of its components.
7 Diagram a skeletal muscle sarcomere, including *actin*, *myosin*, *A band*, *Z line*, *I band*, *H zone*, and *cross bridges*.
8 Describe the mechanical changes in muscle structure during contraction, according to the *sliding-filament model* (see Fig. 10-6, p. 261).
9 Describe and write the three equations that depict the molecular changes in actin, myosin, ADP, and ATP that occur during contraction.
10 Describe the molecular basis for *rigor mortis*.
11 Describe the role of calcium and the role of *regulator proteins*, *troponin*, and *tropomyosin* in contraction.

READING ASSIGNMENT

Chap. 10, pp. 255–264.

EXERCISES

Directions: Answer the following questions in the space provided.

Fig. 10–6, p. 261 1 Diagram the sliding-filament model of muscle contraction and label each element.

262 2 Write the three equations that depict the molecular changes in actin, myosin, ADP, and ATP that occur during contraction.

256 3 Define and differentiate among muscle fiber, myofibrils, and filaments.

263 4 Why might rigor mortis occur more rapidly in an individual who dies during exercise?

SELF-TEST

PART I

Directions: Circle T for true and F for false.

T F 1 Light and dark banding patterns appear on all muscle due to the arrangement of contractile protein.

T F 2 Most smooth muscle is connected to bones.

T F 3 There is a single sarcomere inside each cell which develops the tension for the cell.
T F 4 Muscles are the only cells capable of generating movement.
T F 5 Thick filaments are composed of actin.
T F 6 Each of the filaments in the muscle shortens during contraction.
T F 7 None of the filaments shortens during contraction.
T F 8 Where the filaments overlap, there are twice as many thin filaments as thick filaments.
T F 9 At rest, troponin and tropomyosin inhibit cross-bridge cycling.
T F 10 During a cross-bridge cycle, energy is temporarily stored in the myosin molecule.

PART II

Directions: Complete the following items in the space provided.

1 Three types of muscle can be identified on the basis of structure. They are:

a ____________________

b ____________________

c ____________________

2 The functional unit of the contractile system in striated muscle is the ____________________.

3 The ends of the sarcomere are defined by the ____________ lines.

4 The thick filament is composed of ____________ and the thin filament is composed of ____________.

5 During contraction, the thick and thin filaments are connected by ____________, which generate movement.

6 Calcium binds to the regulator protein ____________, which pulls the ____________ bound to it to one side, uncovering the cross-bridge sites on ____________.

7 ATP provides two distinct functions in the cross-bridge cycle. They are:

a ____________________

b ____________________

8 Tropomyosin and troponin affect myosin ATPase activity by blocking the binding of ____________ to ____________.

9 Tropomyosin and troponin are bound to the ____________ filaments.

Module II • Excitation and contraction of muscle fibers

OBJECTIVES

Upon completion of this module, the student will be able to:

1 Define *excitation-contraction* coupling.
2 Describe the role of calcium in excitation-contraction coupling.
3 Describe the role of the muscle plasma membrane and the *lateral sacs* and *transverse tubules* of the *sarcoplasmic reticulum* in excitation-contraction coupling.
4 List three general ways by which muscle action potentials can be initiated.
5 Describe the anatomical relationships among the *motor neurons*, *motor units*, *motor end plate*, and *neuromuscular junction*.
6 Describe the release, binding, results, and breakdown of *acetylcholine* at the neuromuscular junction.
7 Define muscle *end-plate potential* and describe its relationship to muscle action potential and motor neuron action potential.
8 List four mechanisms by which drugs or disease may interrupt the neuromuscular junction.

READING ASSIGNMENT

Chap. 10, pp. 264–271, including Table 10-1 on p. 272.

EXERCISES

PART I

Directions: Fill in the missing information in the following sequence of events between a nerve action potential and muscle contraction and relaxation.

1 The action potential in the motor neuron causes release at the neuromuscular
268 junction of ________________________________.

268 2 Acetylcholine is bound to reactive sites on the ________________________ membrane.

3 Acetylcholine causes a permeability change, producing a(n) ______________
269 ______________ potential in the muscle membrane.

4 The muscle membrane is depolarized, and the ________________________
269 travels over the entire muscle plasma membrane.

5 Acetylcholine is rapidly destroyed in the end-plate membrane by ____________
270 ____________________.

6 The muscle action potential is propagated from the plasma membrane surface into

the transverse tubules and into the area of the ______________________ of the sarcoplasmic reticulum. 272

7 This depolarization leads to lateral sacs of the sarcoplasmic reticulum surrounding the myofibrils to release ______________________. 272

8 Ca^{2+} binds on the thin actin filament to ______________________. 272

9 This binding releases the inhibition that prevents actin from binding to ______________________. 272

10 $A + M^* \cdot ADP \cdot P_i \rightarrow$ ______________________. 272

11 $A \cdot M^* \cdot ADP \cdot P_i \rightarrow A \cdot M + ADP + P_i$, producing angular movement of ______________________. 272

12 The actin-myosin bond is broken, allowing the cross bridge to relax, when ATP exchanges with ______________________. 272

13 Inhibition of the cross-bridge contraction and relaxation cycles occurs with a drop in the concentration of ______________________. 272

14 The Ca^{2+} level drops as ATP is split and Ca^{2+} returns to the ______________________. 272

PART II

Directions: Draw a figure illustrating the temporal relation between the muscle fiber action potential and the mechanical event of muscle fiber shortening and describe why they are so different. 264–265

SELF-TEST

PART I

Directions: Circle T for true and F for false.

T F 1 Calcium ions are released from the lateral sacs when the t tubules are depolarized.

T F 2 Calcium ions are returned to the lateral sacs by active transport.

T F 3 A motor unit consists of the motor neuron and all the muscle fibers innervated by it.

T F 4 The motor neuron contains an esterase that inactivates acetylcholine following depolarization of the motor end plate.

T F 5 The end-plate potential is the same amplitude as the muscle action potential.

T F 6 There is a one-to-one transmission of an action potential from a motor neuron to a muscle fiber.

T F 7 The action potential in a motor neuron could produce action potentials in several muscle fibers.

PART II

Directions: Complete the following items in the space provided.

1 The action potential that initiates excitation-contraction coupling originates in the muscle plasma membrane adjacent to the ______________________.

2 The junction between nerve fiber and skeletal muscle is known as ______________________.

3 The chemical transmitter agent released at a neuromuscular junction to initiate membrane depolarization of skeletal muscle fiber is ______________________.

4 The cell bodies of the motor neurons are located in the ______________________ and ______________________.

5 The enzyme that degrades acetylcholine is ______________________ and it is located in the specialized membrane of the muscle cell called the ______________________.

6 The combination of the motor neuron and the muscle fibers it innervates is known as a ______________________.

7 Vesicles containing acetylcholine are released into the synaptic cleft from the axon terminal by the process of ______________________.

8 Acetylcholine opens channels in the end-plate membrane that allow the passage of both ______________________ and ______________________ ions.

9 Curare binds to the ______________________ receptor.

10 ______________________ toxin blocks the release of acetylcholine from nerve terminals.

Module III • Muscle mechanics and metabolism

OBJECTIVES

Upon completion of this module, the student will be able to:

1 Define *contraction*, *tension*, and *load*.
2 Differentiate between *isometric* and *isotonic contractions*.
3 Define *latent period* and describe its chemical-mechanical basis.
4 Define *twitch*, *twitch duration*, *contraction time*, *relaxation time*, and *velocity of shortening*.
5 Describe the *frequency-tension relationship* of skeletal muscle by defining *summation*, *tetanus*, *unfused tetanus*, and *fused tetanus*.
6 Define and differentiate between *internal* and *external tension*.
7 Describe the *active state* of a muscle fiber and draw a graph depicting the temporal relation between active state and isometric tension.
8 Describe the *series elastic component* and differentiate it from the contractile component.
9 Define *optimal length* and describe the mechanical factors that lead to a reduction in muscle tension when a muscle is greater or less than optimal length.
10 Graph the relationship between resting muscle length and isometric tension development in skeletal muscle and explain this relationship in terms of the sliding-filament model.
11 Draw a graph depicting the relationship between muscle load and the velocity of shortening.
12 List the three major functions of ATP in the contraction and relaxation of muscle.
13 Identify and diagram the three sources of ATP in active muscle as presented in Fig. 10-25, p. 279.
14 List the three factors that limit the cell's ability to replace ATP by oxidative phosphorylation.
15 Describe the apparent advantages and disadvantages of glycolysis as a means of replacing ATP in active muscle.
16 Describe *muscle efficiency*.
17 Describe *muscle fatigue* and identify the most likely intracellular site to explain this failure in tension development.
18 Define *psychological fatigue*.

READING ASSIGNMENT

Chap. 10, pp. 271–281, review Table 10-1, p. 272.

EXERCISES

Directions: Answer the following questions in the space provided.

1 The resting length at which the muscle can develop the maximum tension is l_0. What are the two factors that lead to decreased tension at shorter or longer rest-
277 ing lengths?

2 Passively stretching a muscle changes the amount of overlap between the thick and thin filaments in the myofibrils. How would the thick and thin filaments look
277 in the following situations?

a at optimal length (l_0)

b at 175 percent of l_0

3 Classic observations and experiments proved the relationship between muscle length and the tension the muscle can develop at that length. Draw a graph to
277 show the following pattern.

a When the muscle is set at a length equal to
60 percent of l_0, it develops no tension.
78 percent of l_0, it develops 78 percent tension.
94 percent of l_0, it develops 100 percent tension.
110 percent of l_0, it develops 100 percent tension.
175 percent of l_0, it develops no tension.

b Shade the band that represents the range of muscle length changes that can occur in the body while the muscles are still attached to bones.

4 ATP plays a central role in muscular activity.
 a Summarize the major sources of ATP in muscle cells. 278–279

___

___

___

 b List the three functions of ATP in muscular activity. 278

___

___

___

SELF-TEST

PART I

Directions: Circle T for true and F for false.

T F 1 In the body where muscles are attached to bones the relaxed length of the muscle is at the minimal length for force generation.

T F 2 The resting length of a muscle determines the amount of isometric tension it can develop.

T F 3 At l_0, which represents the length at which the muscle develops maximum tension, the thick and thin filaments are so far apart that there is no overlap between the two.

T F 4 ATP is necessary for both contraction and relaxation of a muscle.

T F 5 Oxygen must be present for muscles to contract.

T F 6 Creatine phosphate provides the most rapid means of forming ATP in the muscle cell.

T F 7 Total depletion of ATP is the cause for muscle fatigue.

T F 8 Tetanus is the mechanical response to a single action potential.

T F 9 The series elastic element generates approximately one-half the tension during a twitch.

T F 10 External tension increases due to an increase in the amount of time the cross bridges remain active.

PART II

Directions: Complete the following items in the space provided.

1 Oxidative phosphorylation has a limited capacity to replace ATP during exercise due to limited:

 a ______________________,

 b ______________________, and

 c ______________________.

2 The three sources of ATP in muscle are:

a ______________________________,

b ______________________________, and

c ______________________________.

3 The three major functions of ATP in muscle are:

a ______________________________,

b ______________________________, and

c ______________________________.

4 Under anerobic conditions ______________________________ can produce larger quantities of ATP than ______________________________.

5 To produce the same mount of ATP, ______________________________ uses much more glucose than does ______________________________.

6 Phosphorylation of ADP by ______________________________ provides a rapid means of forming ATP at the onset of contractile activity.

7 The series elastic component of muscle plays an important role in ______________ ______________________, which can be either fused or ______________________ ______________.

PART III

Directions: Each of the graphs in Fig. W-6 is characteristic of an isotonic or isometric
twitch. Label each graph as an isotonic or isometric twitch and circle the correct pa-
273 rameter for each (either *tension* or *distance shortened*).

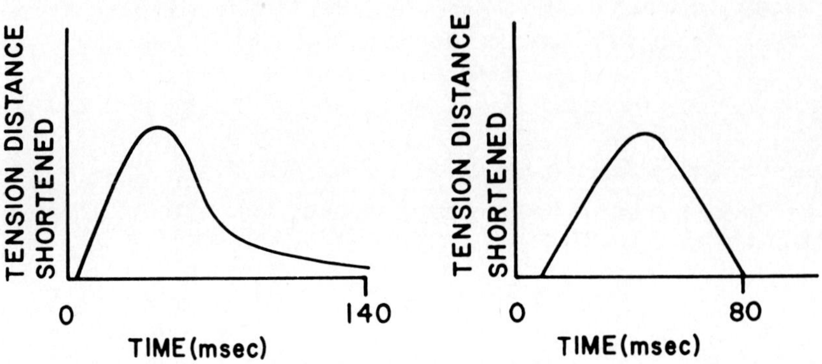

Fig. W-6

Module IV • Characteristics of differentiated muscles

OBJECTIVES

Upon completion of this module, the student will be able to:

1 Describe the differences between an immature *myoblast* and an adult muscle cell.
2 Describe the compensatory mechanisms for loss of muscle in the adult.
3 Define *denervation atrophy*, *disuse atrophy*, and *hypertrophy*.
4 Describe the role of *myoglobin* in determining the color of *red muscle* and *white muscle*.
5 Describe the three types of skeletal muscle that may be distinguished on the basis of ATPase activity and ATP-synthesizing capacity.
6 Describe the role of *tendons* in the transmission of whole-muscle tension.
7 List the factors that determine the *total tension* a muscle can develop.
8 Define *recruitment* and describe its effect on total muscle tension.
9 Compare the changes produced in muscle by high-intensity, short-duration exercise with those produced by low-intensity, long-duration exercise.
10 Differentiate between *flexion* and *extension*.
11 Define *antagonistic muscles*.
12 Define and contrast *concentric* and *eccentric contractions*.
13 Describe how the force exerted by a muscle can be greater than the load it is supporting.
14 Describe how the lever action of muscles improves the maneuverability and velocity of limb movement.
15 List two anatomical characteristics common to all smooth muscle.
16 Describe the cellular anatomy of smooth muscle including a description of *dense bodies*, actin, myosin, and the sliding-filament theory of contraction.
17 Contrast the cellular anatomy of smooth and skeletal muscle.
18 Describe the differences between the excitation-contraction coupling of skeletal and smooth muscle.
19 Describe the role of cytosolic calcium in the maintenance of *tone* in smooth muscle.
20 List five factors that influence smooth muscle contractile activity.
21 Describe the types of *spontaneous electrical activity* found in smooth muscle.
22 Define *varicosities* and differentiate them from the neuromuscular junctions of skeletal muscle.
23 Describe the role of hormones and local factors in the inhibition and excitation of smooth muscle.
24 Describe the classification of smooth muscle on the basis of *single* and *multiunit* smooth muscles.
25 Describe the role of *gap junction* in conduction of electrical activity in smooth and cardiac muscle.

READING ASSIGNMENT

Chap. 10, pp. 281–298.

EXERCISES

Directions: Answer the following questions in the space provided.

281–282 1 Since adult muscle cannot divide to form new cells, how can damage from injury or disease be repaired?

Table 10-2, p. 284 2 List the characteristics of the muscle fibers in an Olympic weight-lifting champion and in a marathon runner and in yourself.

283–288 3 Most of our muscular activity involves smooth and relatively slow muscular contractions. How, then, can the subcellular events described for the twitch be relevant to, e.g., flexion of the arm?

287–289 4 What advantages do tendons and levers have in the transmission of movement from a muscle to a limb?

5 Variability is a key word in describing smooth muscle. Compare and contrast sarcomere organization, dependence on action potentials for contraction, and the neuromuscular junction of smooth muscle with skeletal muscle. **289–295**

____

____

____

SELF-TEST

PART I

Directions: Circle T for true and F for false.

T F 1 Most muscle cells are connected directly to bones.
T F 2 The total tension in a muscle depends both on the number of active fibers and on the tension of each fiber.
T F 3 Increasing the tension in an individual fiber is known as recruitment.
T F 4 Small motor units are associated with fine movements.
T F 5 All the motor units of a given muscle fire at the same time.
T F 6 The tension developed during a twitch defines the maximum tension of that muscle.
T F 7 The force exerted by a muscle is equal to the load it must support.
T F 8 Actin and myosin are present in all three types of muscle.
T F 9 The amount of actin and myosin in a muscle can be changed by exercise.
T F 10 Slow- and fast-twitch fibers differ on the basis of the type of actin and myosin in each fiber.
T F 11 The primary source of ATP is the same for all muscles.
T F 12 A large number of mitochondria are necessary for a muscle to resist fatigue.
T F 13 The sarcoplasmic reticulum is equally well developed in smooth and skeletal muscle.
T F 14 Many smooth muscles undergo continuous low-level contractile activity called tone.
T F 15 Action potentials are necessary for smooth muscle contraction.
T F 16 A given neurotransmitter can be excitatory to one smooth muscle and inhibitory to another smooth muscle.
T F 17 Extracellular calcium can enter a smooth muscle cell and trigger contractile activity.

PART II

Directions: Complete the following items in the space provided.

1 The increase in the size of the individual muscle fibers caused by increased amount of contractile activity is called ____________________.

2 Exercise increases the capacity of a muscle for activity by

a ______

b ______

3 The decrease in muscle mass following denervation is known as what type of atrophy? ______

4 A muscle can atrophy with its nerve supply intact if it is not used for a long time, and this is known as what type of atrophy? ______

5 In a single-unit smooth muscle, the spontaneous depolarization of the membrane that occurs at regular intervals is known as a(n) ______.

6 The shortening of the stronger of two antagonistic muscles is called a ______ contraction.

7 The lengthening of a muscle undergoing active contraction is known as ______ contraction.

8 ______ unit smooth muscles propagate action potentials from fiber to fiber.

9 Stretch induces the contraction of ______ unit smooth muscles.

10 The sarcoplasmic reticulum is most well developed in ______ muscle.

Answers

CHAPTER 10 • MODULE I

PART I

1 F (256)
2 F (255)
3 F (256)
4 F (255)
5 F (256)
6 F (260)
7 T (260)
8 T (260)
9 T (263)
10 T (262)

PART II

1 a skeletal muscle (255)
b smooth muscle (255)
c cardiac muscle (255)
2 sarcomere (256)
3 Z (256)
4 myosin; actin (256)
5 cross bridges (260)
6 troponin; tropomyosin; actin (263–264)
7 a energy for cross-bridge movement (262)
b binding to myosin to break the A-M link (262)
8 actin; myosin (263–264)
9 thin (263)

CHAPTER 10 • MODULE II

PART I

1 T (267)
2 T (267)
3 T (267)
4 F (270)
5 F (269)

6 T (270)
7 T (267, 270)

PART II

1 motor end plate (267)
2 neuromuscular junction (267)
3 acetylcholine (268)
4 brainstem; spinal cord (267)
5 acetylcholine esterase; motor end plate (270)
6 motor unit (267)
7 exocytosis (268)
8 sodium; potassium (269)
9 acetylcholine (271)
10 botulinus (271)

CHAPTER 10 • MODULE III

PART I

1 F (278)
2 T (277)
3 F (277)
4 T (278)
5 F (280)
6 T (279)
7 F (281)
8 F (274–275)
9 F (275–276)
10 T (276)

PART II

1 a O_2 delivery (280)
b nutrient availability (280)
c rate of nutrient metabolism (280)
2 a creatine phosphate (278)
b oxidative phosphorylation (278)
c glycolysis (278)
3 a cross-bridge movement (278)
b breakage of A-M bond (278)
c reaccumlation of calcium ions (278)
4 glycolysis, oxidative phosphorylation (280)
5 glycolysis; oxidative phosphorylation (280)
6 creatine phosphate (279)
7 tetanus; unfused (274–276)

PART III

See Fig. 10-18, p. 273

CHAPTER 10 • MODULE IV

PART I

1 F (284)
2 T (284)
3 F (284)
4 T (285)
5 F (285)
6 F (286)
7 F (289)
8 T (297)
9 T (286)
10 F (283)
11 F (284)
12 T (284)
13 F (297)
14 T (292)
15 F (292)
16 T (295)
17 T (291)

PART II

1 hypertrophy (282)
2 a increase in ATP enzyme-forming capacity (286)
b increase in number myofibrils (286)
3 denervation atrophy (282)
4 disuse atrophy (282)
5 pacemaker or slow wave potential (293)
6 concentric (288)
7 eccentric (288)
8 Single- (296)
9 single- (296)
10 skeletal (297)

11 CIRCULATION

Module I • The blood

OBJECTIVES

Upon completion of this module, the student will be able to:

1 Define in general terms the *circulation* and the *cardiovascular system.*
2 List the three cellular elements and the liquid that make up blood.
3 Define *hematocrit* and state the normal value for men and women.
4 Identify the fractions of body weight represented by *total blood volume, total blood cell volume,* and *total plasma volume.*
5 List the eight electrolytes and three types of *plasma proteins* that are the major components of plasma.
6 State the site of synthesis of the plasma proteins and indicate *immunoglobulins* as the major exception in that they are formed in the lymph nodes.
7 Differentiate between *serum* and *plasma.*
8 Describe the outstanding physical and chemical characteristics of the *erythrocyte.*
9 Describe the basic structure and function of *hemoglobin, heme,* and *globin* in relation to erythrocyte function.
10 Define *sickle-cell anemia.*
11 Describe the life cycle of the erythrocyte indicating the sites of its destruction and the cells involved.
12 Define *erythropoiesis* and its site of occurrence, and define the roles of *iron, vitamin B_{12}, folic acid, heme,* and *globin.*

13 Define *transferrin* and *ferritin*.
14 Define *pernicious anemia*.
15 Describe the origin, site of action, and function of *erythropoietin*.
16 Describe *anemia* and give five general causes of this condition.
17 List the five classes of *leukocytes* and their general function.
18 Define *phagocytosis*.
19 Contrast *mast cells* and *basophils* for appearance, function, and location.
20 State the origin and role of platelets in the blood including the role of the *megakaryocyte* in their formation.

READING ASSIGNMENT

Chap. 11, pp. 302–310.

EXERCISES

Directions: Answer the following questions in the space provided.

1 If red blood cells have an average life expectancy of 120 days, how do we maintain a normal hematocrit? **306–307**

____

____

____

2 What are the general functions that differentiate erythrocytes, leukocytes, and platelets? **304, 309**

____

____

____

3 If bone marrow were destroyed (e.g., by radiation, toxic chemicals, or trauma), what blood cells would be affected and how? **306, 309–310**

____

____

____

SELF-TEST

Directions: Circle T for true and F for false.

T F 1 Blood is a liquid with all its components in solution.
T F 2 Serum is plasma without the red blood cells.

T F 3 In the adult, erythrocytes are produced in the bone marrow, the liver, and the spleen.

T F 4 The average life-span of an erythrocyte is approximately 4 months.

T F 5 Erythrocytes are produced by a process called erythropoietin.

T F 6 Some of the raw materials required to produce erythrocytes are iron, vitamin B_{12}, folic acid, and amino acids.

T F 7 Bilirubin is the component of the hemoglobin molecule with which the oxygen actually combines.

T F 8 Iron balance is maintained by the kidneys alone, whereas vitamin B_{12} is dependent on dietary intake and its balance is maintained by the gastrointestinal system.

T F 9 The erythrocyte lacks a nucleus.

T F 10 Erythropoietin stimulates the production of erythrocytes.

T F 11 Erythropoietin is secreted by the kidney in response to low oxygen delivery.

T F 12 When the erythrocyte dies, the large molecules are broken down by macrophages in the liver, spleen, bone marrow, and lymph nodes.

T F 13 The oxygen-carrying capacity of the erythrocytes is not significantly diminished by the aging of the cell.

Module II • The overall design of the cardiovascular system and heart

OBJECTIVES

Upon completion of this module, the student will be able to:

1 Differentiate between *bulk-flow* and *diffusion.*
2 Differentiate between *pulmonary* and *systemic circulation.*
3 List the vessels that carry blood away from and back to the heart.
4 Define *microcirculation* by listing its components.
5 Describe the unusual connections of the *portal vein.*
6 Define *flow* and state the units used in describing the cardiovascular system.
7 Define *pressure difference* and state the units used in describing the cardiovascular system.
8 Define *resistance* and give the general equation relating it to pressure difference and flow.
9 Define *pericardium* and *myocardium.*
10 List the four chambers of the heart and the four valves of the heart, and state the function of each and the anatomical relationships among them.

11 List the major structures through which blood flows as it passes through the systemic circulation and the pulmonary circulation.
12 Describe the special characteristics of cardiac muscle, including the concepts of *cell length, intercalated discs, desmosomes, gap junctions,* and the *conducting system.*
13 Describe the parts of the heart that are innervated by the sympathetic and parasympathetic nervous system.
14 Define *coronary arteries* and state their function.
15 Define *pacemaker potential* and describe its role in the origin of the heart beat and the major component of its ionic basis.
16 List the sequence of structures and the relative speed of conduction in each for the spread of excitation from the *SA node* to the *ventricular muscle.*
17 Define *electrocardiogram* and its principal elements: *P wave,* the *QRS complex,* and the *T wave,* and the timing of each.
18 List the sequence of events in cardiac *excitation-contraction coupling.*
19 Identify the two sources of calcium in excitation-contraction coupling and indicate their relative contribution to membrane depolarization and cross-bridge activation.
20 Define the *refractory period* of cardiac muscle and describe its critical importance in maintaining cardiac function.
21 Diagram the changes in membrane potential and the mechanical contraction of cardiac muscle and include overall timing and the relative duration of the refractory period.
22 Define *ectopic focus, AV block,* and *ventricular fibrillation.*
23 Define *systole, diastole, end-diastolic volume, end-systolic volume, ventricular ejection,* and *isovolumetric ventricular contraction* and *relaxation.*
24 Diagram and describe the events of the *cardiac cycle* for left side of the heart, including changes in electrocardiogram, heart sounds, chamber pressures, ventricular volume, and valve condition (i.e., reproduce Fig. 11-28, p. 325).
25 Identify the origin of the *lub* and *dub* heart sounds.
26 Define valvular *stenosis* and *regurgitation* and describe the *heart murmurs* associated with these abnormal conditions.
27 Define *cardiac output* and give the equation (including units) to calculate cardiac output from *heart rate* and *stroke volume.*
28 List normal values for cardiac output, heart rate, and stroke volume.
29 Describe the extent and direction to which the autonomic nervous system and automatic mediators alter the spontaneous rhythmic discharge of the SA node.
30 State the ionic basis of the parasympathetic and sympathetic effects on SA nodal pacemaker potential depolarization.
31 Describe and diagram the intrinsic adaptation of the heart to changes in end-diastolic volume (*Starling's law of the heart*).
32 Define *venous return* and state its relationship to Starling's law of the heart.
33 Define *contractility* and identify the effect of sympathetic mechanisms that control stroke volume.

34 Differentiate between the intrinsic and extrinsic mechanisms that control stroke volume.
35 List the factors that increase cardiac output.
36 Describe the determinants of cardiac work and the dissociation between cardiac output and cardiac work.

READING ASSIGNMENT

Chap. 11, pp. 311–332.

EXERCISES

Directions: Answer the following questions in the space provided.

311 1 In an organism the size of a human, what is the adaptive value of a cardiovascular system?

Table 11-3, p. 313 2 State the general function of:

a atria

b ventricles

c arteries

d arterioles

e capillaries

f veins

3 What makes the valves of the heart open and close? What would happen if the AV valves leaked? Would you expect changes in sounds, pressures, and volumes of cardiac chambers? **315, 325–326**

4 Draw and label three beats of a normal electrocardiogram. **321**

5 Why is a specialized conduction system important to the normal functioning of the ventricular myocardium? **319–320**

6 A trained athlete has a maximal cardiac output of 35 L/min. How large an increase in heart rate and/or stroke volume would be necessary to produce this, and how is this increase brought about? **326**

324–325 7 Indicate if the valves are open (O) or closed (C).

Condition	Right AV	Pulmonary	Left AV	Aortic
a isovolumetric contraction	______	______	______	______
b isovolumetric relaxation	______	______	______	______
c middiastole	______	______	______	______
d midsystole	______	______	______	______
e ventricular ejection	______	______	______	______

SELF-TEST

Directions: Circle T for true and F for false.

T F 1 The heart contains special nerves that coordinate the contraction of the heart.

T F 2 The SA node is the only area of the heart capable of developing a pacemaker potential.

T F 3 The AV node delays the conduction of excitation to the ventricles.

T F 4 The inherent autonomous discharge rate of the SA node is greater than the normal resting heart rate.

T F 5 The refractory period of cardiac muscle protects the heart from tetanic contractions.

T F 6 Circulating catecholamines have a major effect on heart rate but no effect on contractility.

T F 7 During isovolumetric ventricular relaxation, all four heart valves are closed.

T F 8 The first heart sound is produced by the closing of the aortic and pulmonary valves.

T F 9 The contraction of the atria is responsible for pumping most of the blood into the ventricles.

T F 10 All the blood in each ventricle is ejected during systole.

T F 11 During systole the aortic valve is closed.

T F 12 Cardiac output can change without a change in heart rate.

T F 13 Stroke volume is the difference between end-diastolic and end-systolic volume.

T F 14 Cardiac work is determined solely by cardiac output.

T F 15 Both interstitial and intracellular calcium are important in cardiac excitation-contraction coupling.

T F 16 Virtually all the blood that goes through the systemic circulation must also go through the right and left side of the heart and the pulmonary circulation.

T F 17 The heart supplies the energy for bulk-flow in both the systemic circulation and pulmonary circulation.

T F 18 The repeated branching of the cardiovascular tree results in relatively small diffusion distances for every cell in the body.

Module III • The vascular system

OBJECTIVES

Upon completion of this module, the student will be able to:

1 Restate from the previous module the equation defining the relation between bulk-flow, pressure difference, and resistance.
2 Describe the relative role of *viscosity, length,* and *radius* of the vessel as each contributes to the resistance in the cardiovascular system.
3 Describe the distinguishing anatomical features of arteries, arterioles, capillaries, veins, and lymphatics.
4 Describe the distinguishing functional characteristics of arteries, arterioles, capillaries, veins, and lymphatics.
5 Describe the "*pressure reservoir*" function of the arteries.
6 Define and give average values for *systolic pressure, diastolic pressure, pulse pressure,* and *mean arterial blood pressure.*
7 Describe the three major factors that determine the pulse pressure.
8 Describe the principle and application of the *sphygmomanometer* in the measurement of blood pressure in humans.
9 Describe the simplifying assumption that allows the statement of the general equation $\text{Flow}_{\text{organ}} = \text{MAP}/\text{Resistance}_{\text{organ}}$.
10 Describe and differentiate between *local controls* and *extrinsic* (reflex) *control* of blood flow to an organ.
11 Define and contrast *active hyperemia* and *pressure autoregulation.*
12 Define and describe the ionic basis of the vascular *myogenic response.*
13 Define *reactive hyperemia.*
14 State the central generalization concerning vasodilation and vasoconstriction of arterioles by the sympathetic nerves.
15 Contrast the role of sympathetic nerves, parasympathetic nerves, and hormones in the extrinsic control of arterioles.
16 Define *metarteriole* and *precapillary sphincter* and distinguish the metarteriole from a true capillary.
17 Describe the two characteristics of the resistance of capillaries that distinguish their resistance from that of arterioles.

18 Describe why the velocity of capillary blood flow is low and the cross-sectional area is high and what the adaptive value of these characteristics is to diffusional exchange.

19 List and describe the role of *capillary hydrostatic pressure, interstitial hydrostatic pressure, plasma protein concentration,* and *interstitial-fluid protein concentration* in the movement of fluid across the capillary wall.

20 Define *capillary absorption, capillary filtration,* and *edema* and the effect of arteriole dilation and constriction on each.

21 Define *central venous pressure* and compare with right atrial pressure.

22 Describe the role of veins as low resistance conduits and blood volume storage vessels (capacity function).

23 Describe the role of venous constriction, the "*skeletal muscle pump,*" and the "*respiratory pump*" in facilitating the return of blood to the heart.

24 Describe the function of valves in the heart, the veins, and the lymphatics in directing lymph or blood flow back to the heart.

25 Describe the four general functions of the lymphatics.

READING ASSIGNMENT

Chap. 11, pp. 332–352.

EXERCISES

Directions: Answer the following questions in the space provided.

1 Explain why arterioles, rather than any other vessel type, are the sites of control
336–337 of resistance in the cardiovascular system.

2 If local controls of blood flow to an organ are so good at matching blood flow to the
needs of the tissue, what might be the point of the apparently redundant "extrin-
339 sic" controls of organ blood flow?

3 A person has severe protein deficiency. Knowing something about the factors con-
trolling net movement of fluid across capillaries, state why these individuals often
348 appear bloated.

4 What would happen to the hematocrit if the lymphatics were allowed to drain outside the body? 351

5 List the four major determinants of venous pressure and describe the direction in which each changes right atrial pressure. 350

6 List the factors that determine pulse pressure. 334

7 Describe the effect of arteriolar vasodilation and vasoconstriction on the factors that determine bulk-flow across the capillary wall. 347

SELF-TEST

Directions: Circle T for true and F for false.

T F 1 The velocity of blood flow is uniform throughout the cardiovascular system.
T F 2 The total cross-sectional area reaches its maximum at the capillaries.
T F 3 The total blood volume can vary during the day because of filtration at the capillaries.
T F 4 All the fluid filtered at the capillaries is returned to the vascular system by the lymphatics.
T F 5 Walking increases the venous return to the heart.
T F 6 The elastic properties of arteries maintain diastolic pressure and flow after the aortic valve has closed.
T F 7 Although the veins are at a lower pressure than the arteries, they still contain a greater portion of the total blood volume.

T F 8 Sympathetic nerve activation can produce constriction in both arteries and veins.

T F 9 The valves in the heart and great veins permit blood flow in only one direction.

T F 10 The magnitude and direction of the hydrostatic pressure head is the sole determinant of filtration or absorption.

T F 11 The pressure drop from the aorta to the wrist artery is small compared with the drop in pressure across the capillaries of the hand.

T F 12 The length and radius are almost equally important in determining resistance in arterioles.

T F 13 Changes in sympathetic nerve activity can produce either vasoconstriction or vasodilation.

T F 14 An increase in stroke volume tends to increase pulse pressure.

T F 15 The radius of a capillary is generally not under active control.

T F 16 Venous constriction decreases the capacitance but has a negligible effect on the resistance in the vein.

T F 17 Lymph vessels connect directly to the venous system.

T F 18 The "skeletal muscle pump" and the "respiratory pump" work to move fluid in one direction in either veins and lymphatics.

T F 19 Protein and electrolytes are filtered across the capillary membrane into the interstitial fluid space in a concentration equal to that found in plasma.

T F 20 The same hormone can be a vasoconstrictor in one vascular bed and a vasodilator in another.

Module IV • Regulation of the cardiovascular system in health and disease

OBJECTIVES

Upon completion of this module, the student will be able to:

1 List the six basic components of a reflex control system.
2 State the major variable regulated by the cardiovascular system and indicate its relation to cardiac output and the resistance to flow offered by the vascular system.
3 Define *total peripheral resistance* (TPR) and identify the relative importance of different vessel types to TPR.
4 Develop the equation: Mean arterial blood pressure = cardiac output × TPR from the general bulk-flow equation. List and justify each assumption.
5 Define *baroreceptor* and indicate the two primary arterial baroreceptor areas.

6 Describe the arterial *baroreceptor reflex arc* and include the concepts of sensitivity to mean and pulsatile pressure.
7 Describe the general function of baroreceptors other than those of the carotid sinus and aortic arch.
8 Describe the *medullary cardiovascular center's* role in blood pressure regulation by listing the four general efferent activities initiated in response to a decrease in arterial pressure.
9 Describe the input to the medullary cardiovascular center from neurons in the hypothalamus, cortex, and other brain areas.
10 Define *hypotension* and indicate that blood or fluid loss, decreased sympathetic nerve activity, and increased parasympathetic nerve activity are the three general causes for this condition.
11 Describe the reflexes that occur via the medullary cardiovascular center during hypotension.
12 Describe the compensatory changes between capillary fluid and interstitial fluid that occur during hypotension.
13 List the direction of change in total blood volume, erythrocyte volume, plasma volume, and plasma albumin that occur immediately after hemorrhage and 18 h following the hemorrhage.
14 Define *circulatory shock* and identify conditions under which it becomes irreversible.
15 Describe the cardiovascular compensations caused by getting out of bed and standing upright.
16 Describe the cardiac and peripheral vascular responses to exercise.
17 Describe the effect of endurance exercise training on cardiovascular function.
18 Define *hypertension, renal hypertension,* and *primary hypertension* and indicate the primary defect responsible for these conditions.
19 Define and identify the symptoms and cardiovascular defects associated with *congestive heart failure, pulmonary edema, myocardial infarction, atherosclerosis, angina pectoris,* and *stroke.*

READING ASSIGNMENT

Chap. 11, pp. 352–371

EXERCISES

Directions: Answer the following questions in the space provided.

1 List the sensor, afferent limb, integrator, efferent limb, and effectors in the arterial baroreceptor reflex. **355–358**

____

____

____

2 What can you say about the resistance to blood flow in the pulmonary vasculature (compared with TPR), knowing that the pulmonary arterial pressure is considerably lower than the mean arterial pressure of systemic arteries? 352–353

3 Describe the compensatory reflexes and alterations in fluid exchange that occur during hemorrhage. 362–363

365–367 4 What happens to mean arterial pressure during exercise? Why?

5 Describe how a transplanted (i.e., totally denervated) heart can respond to the body's needs during exercise. Consider the discussion of the importance of venous return to promoting cardiac output. 367

370–371 6 How might a myocardial infarction lead to death?

369 7 What is the major abnormality in hypertension?

370 8 Why might individuals with congestive heart failure "drown" in their own fluid?

SELF-TEST

PART I

Directions: Circle the correct answer(s).

1 Concerning total peripheral resistance, which of the following are true?
  a The average radius of the arterioles is the single most important determinant of TPR.
  b TPR can be calculated from heart rate and stroke volume.
  c The pulmonary circulation is not included in TPR.
  d Both local and autonomic control mechanisms can alter TPR.
  e TPR is reflexly increased in response to hemorrhage.

2 Concerning severe hemorrhage, which of the following are true?
  a Reflex adjustments include an increase in venous constriction.
  b A decrease in interstitial-fluid volume can occur in response to hemorrhage.
  c Initially the hemorrhage results in a decreased firing of the baroreceptors.
  d Both heart rate and stroke volume are reflexly increased.
  e Plasma volume remains below normal for several days.

3 Concerning hypotension, which of the following are true?
  a Hypotension can occur even when cardiac output is very high, for example when TPR is very low.
  b Hypotension can occur even with a normal blood volume.
  c Irreversible shock can occur even if blood volume is returned to normal.
  d Hypotension is generally associated with the decrease in TPR that occurs with exercise.
  e The initial response to the upright posture is similar to the initial response to hypotension.

PART II

Directions: Complete the schematic of the basic reflex regulation of arterial blood pressure that is shown in figure W-7 on page 128.

Module V • Hemostasis

OBJECTIVES

Upon completion of this module, the student will be able to:

1 Define and state the two basic prerequisites for *hemorrhage.*
2 Define *hemostasis.*
3 Define *hematoma.*

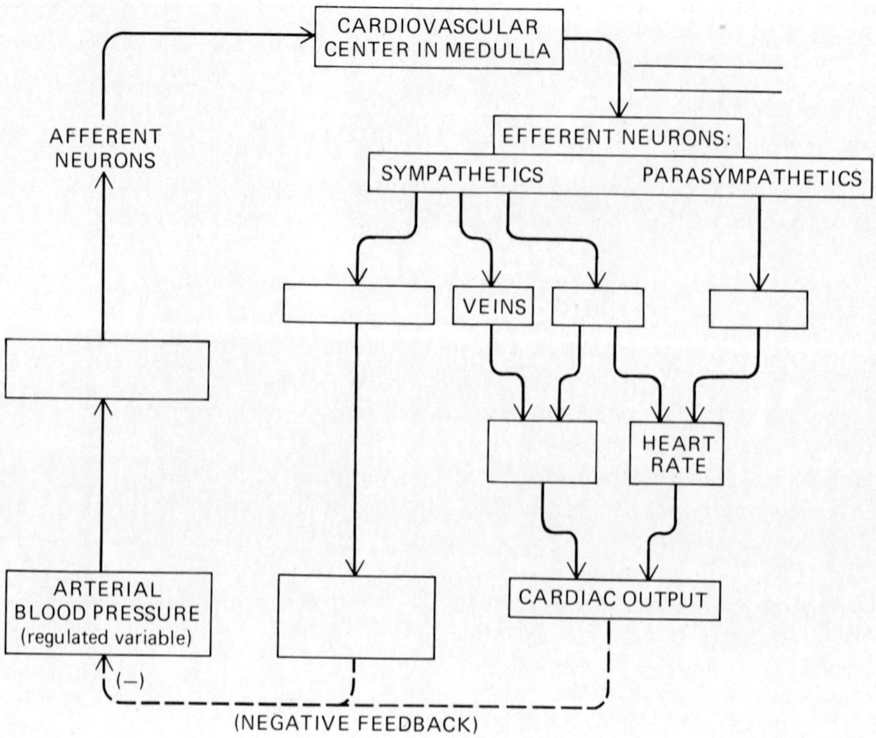

Fig. W-7

4 State why venous and small-vessel bleeding is less serious than large-vessel and arterial bleeding.
5 Describe the four critical roles of platelets in hemostasis as *adherence* to collagen, *aggregation* to form plug, *secretion* of platelet granules, and platelet *contraction.*
6 State the general relation among fibrinogen, thrombin, and fibrin.
7 Diagram and state the general principle of the *cascade* theory of clotting.
8 Identify the role of *factor XIII, prothrombin, and factor XII* (*Hageman factor*) in the generation of fibrin.
9 Define *hemophilia.*
10 Describe the role played by the liver in the overall functioning of the clotting mechanism.
11 Differentiate between the *extrinsic* and *intrinsic clotting pathways* by identifying the role of *tissue thromboplastin* in the clotting mechanism.
12 Describe the role of *plasmin* and *plasminogen* in the process of dissolving a clot.
13 Describe the anticoagulant activity of plasmin and *heparin.*
14 Define intravascular *thrombosis, hypercoagulability, emboli,* and *thrombus.*

READING ASSIGNMENT

Chap. 11, pp. 372–378.

EXERCISES

Directions: Answer the following questions in the space provided.

1 List the four hemostatic events involving platelets. **372–373**

2 Diagram the general relation among fibrinogen, thrombin, and fibrin in the process of blood clotting. **374**

3 Describe why plasminogen and heparin are critically important to the normal operation of the cardiovascular system. **377**

4 Describe what is meant by "amplification" in the clotting cascade. **375–376**

5 List the components of the clotting system that are synthesized by the liver. **376**

SELF-TEST

Directions: Circle T for true and F for false.

T F 1 The formation of a fibrin clot is a single enzymatic reaction.
T F 2 Platelets adhere to normal endothelial cells.
T F 3 Aggregated platelets release powerful vasoconstrictors.
T F 4 Two naturally occurring anticoagulants are plasmin and thrombin.

T F 5 Most of the enzymes in the clotting cascade are present in an inactive form in normal blood.

T F 6 Contact with the damaged vessel surface is the trigger for the clotting cascade.

T F 7 One or more of the factors can be missing from the cascade and clotting will proceed normally.

T F 8 Tissue thromboplastin can initiate clot formation by the extrinsic clotting pathway.

Answers

CHAPTER 11 • MODULE I

1 F	(302)
2 F	(303)
3 F	(306)
4 T	(306)
5 F	(307)
6 T	(306–307)
7 F	(305)
8 F	(306–307)
9 T	(305)
10 T	(307)
11 T	(307)
12 T	(306)
13 T	(306)

CHAPTER 11 • MODULE II

1 F	(317)
2 F	(319)
3 T	(319)
4 T	(327)
5 T	(322)
6 F	(331)
7 T	(324–325)
8 F	(326)
9 F	(324)
10 F	(324)
11 F	(325–326)
12 T	(326)
13 T	(324, 326)
14 F	(331)
15 T	(322)
16 T	(311)
17 T	(311)
18 T	(311)

CHAPTER 11 • MODULE III

1 F	(342–343)
2 T	(342–343)
3 T	(351)
4 F	(347)
5 T	(350)
6 T	(333)
7 T	(349)
8 T	(339, 349)
9 T	(351)
10 F	(347)
11 T	(332)
12 F	(332)
13 T	(339)
14 T	(334)
15 T	(342)
16 T	(349)
17 T	(351)
18 T	(350–351)
19 F	(346)
20 T	(340)

CHAPTER 11 • MODULE IV

PART I

1 a, c, d, e	(352–354, 362–363)
2 a, b, c, d	(362–363)
3 a, b, c, e	(362–364)

PART II

See Fig. 11-63, p. 358

CHAPTER 11 • MODULE V

1 F	(373–376)
2 F	(373)
3 T	(373)
4 F	(377)
5 T	(374)
6 T	(372)
7 F	(375)
8 T	(376)

12
RESPIRATION

Module I • Basic structure and function of the respiratory system
Module II • Exchange and transport of gases in the body
Module III • Control of respiration

Module I • Basic structure and function of the respiratory system

OBJECTIVES

Upon completion of this module, the student will be able to:

1 Define *respiration* (two meanings), *respiratory system, ventilation*, and *gas exchange*.
2 Label the following structures on diagrams of the respiratory system and identify the function of each: nasal passage, oral cavity, pharynx, larynx, trachea, bronchi, diaphragm, lungs (various lobes), pleura, alveoli, and bronchioles.
3 Describe the four major functions, in addition to air flow, of the *conducting portions* of the respiratory system including the function of the *cilia* and the *vocal cords*.
4 Describe how the structure of the alveoli is well adapted to the exchange of gases across their walls.
5 Describe and state the importance of *collateral ventilation*.
6 Describe the general structure of the *thoracic cage* including the terms diaphragm, sternum, ribs, and intercostal muscles.
7 Describe the relationship of the lungs to the thoracic cage including a description of the *pleura* and the *intrapleural fluid*.
8 Define and compare *intrapleural air pressure* and *alveolar air pressure*.
9 Define *pneumothorax* and its effects on the lungs.
10 Define *intrathoracic pressure*.
11 List and describe the four major steps involved in respiration.

12 Write the equation for bulk-flow and define each term as it applies to the respiratory system.
13 Define *inspiration* and *expiration.*
14 Diagram the changes in intrapleural and alveolar pressures during a normal and during a forced inspiration and expiration (see Fig. 12-11, p. 388, and Fig. 12-13, p. 390).
15 Define and describe *lung compliance.*
16 Define alveolar *surface tension* and the effects of *pulmonary surfactant* on total lung compliance.
17 Describe the *respiratory-distress syndrome* of the newborn.
18 Define *airway resistance* and list the factors that determine airway resistance.
19 List the neural and chemical factors that constrict and dilate the airways.
20 Describe the *Heimlich* maneuver in terms of the pressure and volume changes in the respiratory system.
21 Identify and give approximate normal values for *inspiratory reserve volume, tidal volume, expiratory reserve volume, residual volume,* and *total lung volume* as measured by a spirograph (see Fig. 12-15, p. 393).
22 Identify and give approximate normal values for *vital capacity, inspiratory capacity,* and *functional residual capacity.*
23 Define *total pulmonary ventilation.*
24 Define *anatomic dead space* and *alveolar dead space.*
25 Define *alveolar ventilation.*
26 Differentiate and calculate, given appropriate data, total pulmonary ventilation and alveolar ventilation.
27 Define and describe *alveolar dead space* and *total (physiological) dead space.*
28 Describe the determinants of the work of breathing.

READING ASSIGNMENT

Chap. 12, pp. 379–394.

EXERCISES

Directions: Answer the following questions in the space provided.

379 1 A unicellular organism can exchange gases with the atmosphere. Why, then, is the complex respiratory system of the human necessary for gas exchange with the atmosphere.

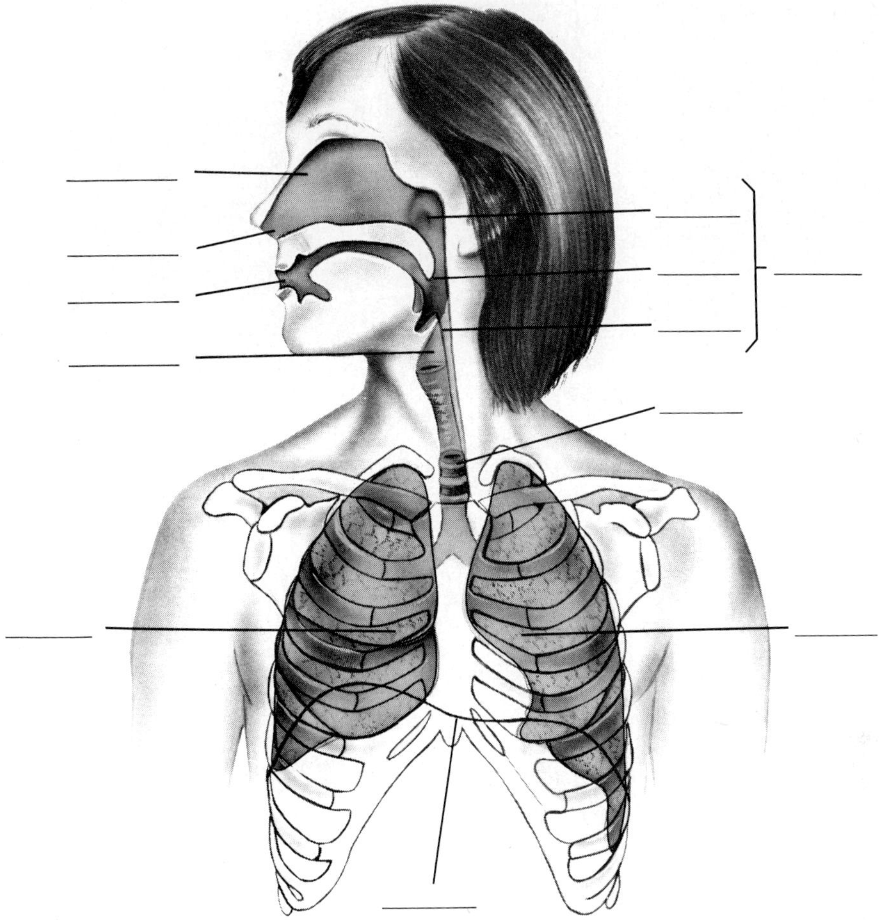

Fig. W-8: Respiratory system.

2 Label the Fig. W-8 and state the function of each labeled part. **Fig. 12-1, p. 380**

3 Describe the *Heimlich* maneuver in terms of the pressure and volume changes in the respiratory system. **391**

____

____

____

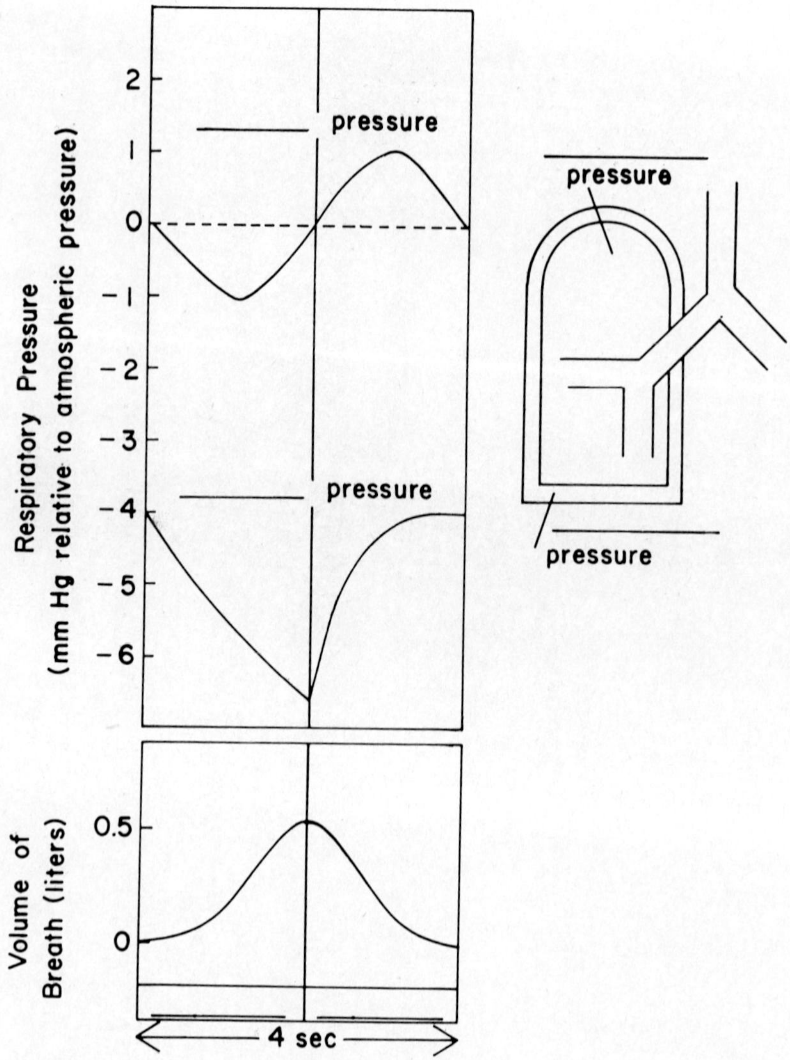

Fig. W-9: Pressure changes during respiration.

3 Fill in the labels on Fig. W-9, indicating the specific types of pressure. You can
388 check your answers against Fig. 12-11, p. 388.

4 Complete Charts 1 and 2 to calculate alveolar ventilation. Use 150 mL as the volume for the dead-space volume. In Chart 2 use the frequency and volumes given in Chart 1 to calculate the dead-space ventilation. You can check your calculations
393 for entries A, C, and D with Table 12-2, p. 393.

Chart 1

Subject	Tidal Volume (mL/breath)	*	Frequency (breaths/min) =	Total Pulmonary Ventilation (mL/min)
A	150	*	40 =	________
B	250	*	24 =	________
C	500	*	12 =	________
D	1000	*	6 =	________

In Chart 2 use the values calculated in Chart 1 for the total pulmonary ventilation for subjects A through D. Again use 150 mL as the dead-space value and the frequency of respiration provided above.

Chart 2

Subject	Total Pulmonary Ventilation (mL/min)−		Dead-Space Ventilation (dead-space vol. × frequency, mL/breath × breath/min) (mL/min)	=	Alveolar Ventilation (mL/min)
A	________	−	________	=	0
B	6000	−	(150) × (24)	=	________
C	________	−	________	=	4200
D	________	−	900	=	5100

6 Draw an idealized spirograph tracing of inspiratory reserve volume, tidal volume, expiratory reserve volume, residual volume, and total lung volume as measured by a spirograph.

Fig. 12–15, p. 393

SELF-TEST

PART I

Directions: Circle T for true and F for false.

T F 1 The cilia are found in the pleura, near the alveoli.
T F 2 The cilia are hairlike projections on the epithelial linings of the alveoli.
T F 3 The cilia help move mucus along the air passages toward the pharynx.
T F 4 The conducting airways cannot exchange gas, and their volume is called the alveolar dead space.
T F 5 Two factors closely related to the "work of breathing" are the stretchability of the lungs and the amount of airway resistance.
T F 6 Pneumothorax aids in alveolar ventilation.
T F 7 Asthma causes a dilation of the airways and an increase in the anatomic dead space.
T F 8 Collateral ventilation is the flow of air through pores between adjacent alveoli.

PART II

Directions: This exercise will take you through the steps in respiration. Answer the questions in order, as many depend on previous responses. Circle the correct answer(s) or fill in the spaces.

1 No air is flowing; all respiratory muscles are relaxed. The subject is in the stage
  a of inspiration.
  b at the end of inspiration prior to expiration.
  c of expiration.
  d at the end of expiration and prior to inspiration.
2 The intrapleural pressure at rest is
  a atmospheric. b subatmospheric. c greater than atmospheric.
3 The intraalveolar pressure at rest is
  a atmospheric. b subatmospheric. c greater than atmospheric.
4 At this point, inspiration is initiated. The first step is
  a contraction of the alveoli.
  b simultaneous contraction of the diaphragm and intercostal muscles, causing an enlargement of the chest cavity.
  c an increase in intrapleural pressure.
5 When the intrapleural pressure becomes even more subatmospheric, what effect does it have on the intraalveolar pressure? ______________________________

____

6 The result of the dropping of intraalveolar pressure below atmospheric pressure is

____.

7 At the end of inspiration, the intraalveolar pressure is ______________________

and the intrapleural pressure is ______________________________.

8 Expiration is initiated by relaxation of what muscle(s)? ______________________

____

9 What effect does the decrease in size of the thoracic cavity have on the intrapleural pressure? ______________________________

____

10 What effect does the decrease in size of the thoracic cavity have on the intraalveolar pressure? ______________________________

____

11 What is the net result of the increase in intrapleural pressure and the intraalveolar pressure? ______________________________

____

PART III

Directions: Write in the term or phrase that completes each definition or example below.

1 Air in the intrapleural space is a ______________________________.

2 Pressure that is always subatmospheric during normal breathing is ______________________________.

3 Movement of air into or out of the lungs is ______________________________.

4 Total amount of air that can be moved in and out during a single breath is ______________________________.

5 Volume of air in lungs after a forceful expiration is ______________________________.

6 Volume of air breathed into or out of the lungs in a normal breath is ______________________________.

7 Volume of air that can be breathed out after a normal expiration is ______________________________.

8 Volume of air that can be breathed in after a normal inspiration is ______________________________.

9 Sum of tidal, inspiratory reserve, and expiratory reserve volume is ______________________________.

10 The phospholipid lining of the alveoli is ______________________________.

11 Tidal volume times the number of respirations per minute is called ______________________________.

12 Alveolar ventilation is calculated as the frequency of breathing times (tidal volume minus ______________________________).

13 If your inspiratory reserve volume is 300 mL, your expiratory reserve volume is 400 mL, and your vital capacity is 1800 mL, how much air do you normally breathe in or out in a single breath while resting? ______.

14 The volume of air still remaining in the lungs after a maximal expiration is the ____________________; its approximate normal value is ______ mL.

15 The amount of air that can be inspired or expired beyond the resting tidal volume is the inspiratory or expiratory ____________________. The normal volumes, respectively, are approximately ______ and ______ mL.

16 The volume of air entering or leaving the lungs in a single breath is the ____________________; its normal resting volume is approximately ______ mL.

17 Those structures that are concerned with the exchange of gas between the blood and the external environment are collectively called the ____________________.

18 The exchange of air between the atmosphere and the alveoli is called ____________________.

19 The exchange of gas between the cells of the body and the external environment is called ____________________.

Module II • Exchange and transport of gases in the body

OBJECTIVES

Upon completion of this module, the student will be able to:

1 Define *respiratory quotient* and state, as examples, the RQs of glucose and fat.
2 State the normal values for oxygen consumed and carbon dioxide produced by man at rest.
3 Define gas pressure in terms of gas concentration and temperature.
4 Define *partial pressure* of a gas and differentiate it from total pressure.
5 Describe the determinants of gas concentrations in a liquid.
6 State the two major determinants of alveolar gas pressures.
7 Define *hyperventilation* and *hypoventilation* and state what effects they have on alveolar gas partial pressures.
8 Describe alveolar-blood gas exchange and the effect of *emphysema, pneumonia,* and *beryllium* on this diffusion process.
9 Describe the control of pulmonary arterioles and bronchioles by local oxygen and carbon dioxide partial pressures.
10 Describe how bronchiolar smooth muscle dilation or constriction and pulmonary arteriolar dilation or constriction produce a matching of ventilation and blood flow in the alveolus.

11 Describe the partial-pressure gradients for oxygen and carbon dioxide from the atmosphere to the tissue and back again.
12 Specify the two forms in which oxygen is carred in the blood and the approximate percentages of oxygen carried in each form.
13 Define *hemoglobin, oxyhemoglobin, deoxyhemoglobin* (or reduced hemoglobin); describe the role of each in the transport of oxygen in the blood.
14 Define *hemoglobin saturation* and draw the *oxygen-hemoglobin dissociation* (or *saturation) curve*.
15 Differentiate among partial pressure of oxygen, total quantity of oxygen, and percent saturation of hemoglobin in the blood.
16 Describe the effect of acidity, temperature, and DPG on the oxygen-hemoglobin dissociation curve and describe the adaptive value of each effect.
17 Name the functions served by *carbonic anhydrase* in gas transport.
18 List the three forms in which carbon dioxide is carried in the blood and the approximate percentage of carbon dioxide carried in each form.
19 Describe the relation between gas and hydrogen-ion transport in blood by drawing the equations for the buffering of hydrogen ion by hemoglobin.

READING ASSIGNMENT

Chap. 12, pp. 394–408.

EXERCISES

PART I

Directions: Complete the following items in the space provided.

1 Assume that your respiratory system produces 8 molecules of carbon dioxide for every 10 molecules of oxygen consumed. What is your respiratory quotient?

______________________ What would be the RQ if pure glucose were used for energy? ______________________ If pure fat were used?

______________________ 395

2 Assume atmospheric pressure at sea level is 760 mmHg. If air contains 21 percent oxygen, what is the partial pressure of oxygen ($P\text{O}_2$) at sea level? ______________

3 Refer to Fig. 12-17, p. 397, to answer these questions.

a $P\text{O}_2$ is highest in the ______________________. 396

b Except in the cells, $P\text{O}_2$ is lowest in the ______________________.

c Except in the cells, $P\text{O}_2$ is highest in the ______________________.

d $P\text{CO}_2$ is lowest in the ______________________.

e In alveolar air, $P\text{CO}_2$ is (greater than, equal to, or less than) the $P\text{CO}_2$ of inspired air. ______________________

f In alveolar air, $P\text{O}_2$ is (greater than, equal to, or less than) the $P\text{O}_2$ of inspired air. ______________________

4 List in order five steps in carbon dioxide exchange between cells and alveoli.

406 a ________________ d ________________

b ________________ e ________________

c ________________

5 Oxygen in the blood can be carried in two ways.

a Combined with hemoglobin b Dissolved in the blood

401–402 The percentage saturation refers to which of these? ________________

6 The approximate percentages of carbon dioxide physically dissolved is ________________, in the form of HCO_3^- is ________________

406 and in the form of $HbCO_2$ is ________________.

PART II

1 Directions: Arrange these steps in order. Enter the number of the step (1,2, etc.)

404 in the space provided.

___O_2 enters pulmonary capillaries. ___O_2 crosses cell membrane.

___O_2 leaves tissue capillaries. ___O_2 is transported in the bloodstream.

___O_2 crosses alveolar membrane.

2 Describe why increased temperature, hydrogen-ion concentration, and DPG levels

404–405 in an exercising muscle are beneficial.

____

____

____

3 Describe how local P_{O_2} affects pulmonary arterioles and contrast this effect with the effect on systemic arterioles. Identify the adaptive value of these differing ef-

399–400 fects.

____

____

____

4 What is the physiological importance of matching ventilation and blood flow to the

399–400 alveolus?

____

____

____

Fig. 12-18, p. 398 5 Diagram the difference in the effect of hypoventilation and hyperventilation on the partial pressure of oxygen and carbon dioxide in alveolar gas.

SELF-TEST

PART I

Directions: Complete the following items in the space provided.

1 Write the equation for the respiratory quotient (RQ). RQ = ____.

2 What is the respiratory quotient for glucose? ______ For fat? ______

3 The pressure of a gas is proportional to its ______________________ and ______________________.

4 The movement of molecules from an area of high concentration to an area of low concentration usually occurs passively by ______________________.

5 The amount of oxygen entering a liquid from a gas is a function of ______________________ and the ______________________.

6 Name the forms in which oxygen is carried in the blood and give the approximate percentage of oxygen carried in each form.

a ______________________ ______%.

b ______________________ ______%.

7 Name the three forms in which carbon dioxide is carred in the blood and give the approximate percentage of carbon dioxide carried in each form.

a ______________________ ______%

b ______________________ ______%

c ______________________ ______%

8 What catalyst facilities the reaction:

$CO_2 + H_2O \rightleftharpoons H_2CO_3$? ______________________

9 What are the two ions formed from carbonic acid?

a ______________________ b ______________________

10 The percentage hemoglobin saturated by oxygen is affected by
a $P\text{CO}_2$. b temperature. c acidity. d $P\text{O}_2$.

PART II

Directions: The symbols > (greater than) and < (less than) are used to show a relationship between two quantities. Insert the appropriate symbol between the values below.

1 $P\text{O}_2$ in inspired air ______ $P\text{O}_2$ in alveolar air.

2 $P\text{O}_2$ in alveolar air ______ $P\text{O}_2$ in pulmonary arteries and systemic veins.

3 $P\text{O}_2$ in tissues ______ $P\text{O}_2$ in pulmonary veins and systemic arteries.

4 $P\text{CO}_2$ in inspired air ______ $P\text{CO}_2$ in alveolar air.

5 $P\text{CO}_2$ in alveolar air ______ $P\text{CO}_2$ in pulmonary arteries and systemic veins.

6 $P\text{CO}_2$ in tissues ______ $P\text{CO}_2$ in pulmonary veins and systemic arteries.

Module III • Control of respiration

OBJECTIVES

Upon completion of this module, the student will be able to:

1 Identify the anatomic site responsible for the rhythmic pattern of breathing.
2 Define *inspiratory neuron* and describe the current model to explain the on-off cycle of their output.
3 Describe the effect of synaptic input to the *medullary respiratory center* from the *pons* and the *pulmonary stretch receptors.*
4 Name and locate the peripheral (the *carotid* and *aortic bodies*) and central *chemoreceptors.*
5 Differentiate between the chemical sensitivities of the peripheral and central chemoreceptor for oxygen, carbon dioxide, and hydrogen ion.
6 Compare and contrast the effects of arterial oxygen, carbon dioxide, and hydrogen on ventilation.
7 Identify the characteristic changes in ventilation during exercise and give the reasons why the stimuli of decreased oxygen or increased carbon dioxide and hydrogen ion do not adequately account for these changes.
8 State the multiple factors that are thought to affect ventilation during exercise.
9 Describe the protective reflexes of coughing and sneezing and how they alter normal ventilatory patterns.
10 Describe the interaction between involuntary and voluntary control of breathing.
11 Define *sleep apnea* and describe its possible role in the *sudden-infant-death* syndrome.
12 Define and differentiate among *hypoxic hypoxia, anemic hypoxia, ischemic hypoxia*, and *histotoxic hypoxia.*
13 Define *mountain sickness* by describing its cause and symptoms.
14 Describe the four major compensations in response to high-altitude hypoxia.
15 Describe and give examples of the metabolic functions of the lungs.

READING ASSIGNMENT

Chap. 12, pp. 408–420.

EXERCISES

PART I

Directions: Answer the following questions in the space provided.

1 Cardiac muscle and the diaphragm both contract rhythmically. What is the fun-
408 damental difference in the origin of the rhythmic activity in these two muscles?

2 The only function of the systems that control respiratory musculature is the maintenance of adequate gas exchange. Defend or refute this statement. **416–417**

3 Defend the position that you could die from hypoxia even with a normal arterial P_{O_2}. **417**

4 What is meant by metabolic functions of the lungs? **419–420**

5 Draw the line graphs indicating the relation between arterial P_{O_2}, P_{CO_2}, and hydrogen-ion concentration and ventilation. On each graph indicate the normal gas partial pressure or hydrogen-ion concentration. In checking your answer be sure to notice the units on each axis. **410–411, 414**

PART II

Directions: Complete the following items in the space provided.

1 When one inhales carbon monoxide, the ventilatory rate does not increase significantly, even though death may ensure from oxygen lack. Why is it that the oxygen lack does not increase the breathing rate and depth? **411**

2 Suppose you are performing an experiment in which the subject hyperventilates for 5 min. Then you ask the subject to relax and just breathe normally (this was 17 breaths/min before hyperventilation). What would you expect to happen to the breathing rate? ______

412 ______

412 What receptors would be affected? ______

What would happen during the hyperventilation, and afterward to arterial P_{O_2}?

______

______

______

398 ______

SELF-TEST

PART I

Directions: Circle the correct answer(s).

1 There remains some controversy about the factors causing the rhythmic firing of the inspiratory neurons in the brainstem. Your textbook supports which of the following views?
   a These neurons cycle in a self-cycling circuit.
   b These neurons have important synaptic input from other brain centers.
   c Both (a) and (b).
   d Neither (a) nor (b).

2 The medullary inspiratory neurons receive inputs from which of the following?
   a feedback connections with the medullary inspiratory neurons
   b connections with higher brain centers
   c connections with the pons
   d carotid sinus and aortic arch
   e stretch receptors in the lungs

3 Which of the following conditions reduce the oxygen content of the blood without concurrently dropping partial pressure of oxygen in the blood?
   a histotoxic hypoxia
   b anemia
   c emphysema
   d carbon monoxide poisoning
   e asthma

4 The respiratory rate is most readily increased by a
   a low P_{O_2} in inspired air.
   b high P_{CO_2} in inspired air.
   c lowering of body temperature.
   d decrease in hydrogen-ion concentration in the blood.

5 The concentration of H^+ in which of the following locations has the greatest influence on respiration?
 a tissues
 b blood
 c alveoli
 d cerebrospinal fluid
 e kidneys
6 Which of the following has been identified as the major variable contributing to the ventilation changes during exercise?
 a P_{CO_2}
 b P_{O_2}
 c H^+ concentration
 d temperature
 e none of the above
7 When an individual is involved in heavy exercise, the alveolar ventilation is increased 10 to 20 times. Which of the following are true of the heavy exercise?
 a Anatomic dead space decreases.
 b Arterial P_{O_2} is drastically reduced.
 c Arterial P_{CO_2} is elevated.
 d The chemical changes in the blood do not fully explain the ventilation pattern.
8 Hypoxia is present when
 a mitochondria are poisoned by cyanide.
 b arteriolar vasoconstriction reduces blood flow below that required by the tissue.
 c following hemorrhage,the hematocrit is drastically reduced.
 d the P_{O_2} of the arterial blood is reduced.
 e any of the above occur.
9 In response to high altitude
 a alveolar ventilation increases.
 b hematocrit increases.
 c muscle myoglobin increases.
 d tissue mitochondria increase.
 e pulmonary vascular resistance increases.
 f all of the above occur.

PART II

Directions: Complete the following items in the space provided.

1 Two receptors for the partial pressure of oxygen are

 a ______________________________

 b ______________________________

2 An increase in H-ion concentration (increases/decreases) ______________ the rate of inspiratory neuron firing, whereas a decrease in H-ion concentration (increases/decreases) ______________________the rate of firing.

3 Exaggerated depression of ventilation during sleep is called ________________.

4 Central chemoreceptors respond to ________________.

5 Abnormal ventilation and blood flow in the lungs produce what form of hypoxia? ________________

6 Exposure to high altitude causes what kind of hypoxia? ________________

Answers

CHAPTER 12 • MODULE I

PART I

1 F (382)
2 F (383)
3 T (382)
4 F (392)
5 T (394)
6 F (385–386)
7 F (390)
8 T (383)

PART II

1 d (387)
2 b (385)
3 a (385)
4 b (387)
5 reduces it below atmospheric (387–388)
6 a pressure gradient for bulk-flow from atmosphere to alveoli (388)
7 atmospheric; more subatmospheric than at rest (388)
8 inspiratory muscles or diaphragm and intercostal muscles (387–388)
9 raises it toward atmospheric pressure or above if forced (388, 390)
10 intraalveolar pressure increases but returns to atmospheric at rest (388)
11 bulk-flow from alveoli to atmosphere (388)

PART III

1 pneumothorax (386)
2 intrapleural (388)
3 bulk-flow or ventilation (386)
4 vital capacity (391)
5 residual volume (391)
6 tidal volume (391)
7 expiratory reserve volume (391)
8 inspiratory reserve volume (391)
9 vital capacity (391)
10 pulmonary surfactant (389)
11 total pulmonary ventilation (392)
12 dead-space volume (393)
13 1100 mL (391, 393)
14 residual volume; 1000 (391, 393)
15 reserve volume; 3000; 1000 (391, 393)
16 tidal volume, 500 (391)
17 respiratory system (380)
18 ventilation (386)
19 respiration (379)

CHAPTER 12 • MODULE II

PART I

1 CO_2 produced/O_2 consumed (395)
2 1.0, 0.7 (395)
3 concentration, speed of molecules (or temperature) (396)
4 diffusion (399)
5 P_{O_2} in gas, solubility of O_2 in liquid (396–397)
6 a Dissolved, approx. 2 (401)
  b Bound to hemoglobin, approx. 98 (401)
7 a Dissolved, approx. 10 (406)
  b Bound to hemoglobin, approx. 30 (406)
  c As bicarbonate, approx. 60 (406)
8 carbonic anhydrase (405)
9 a hydrogen ions (405)
  b bicarbonate ions (405)
10 a, b, c, d (404–407)

PART II

1 > (397)
2 > (397)
3 < (397)
4 < (397)
5 < (397)
6 > (397)

CHAPTER 12 • MODULE III

PART I

1 c (409)
2 a, b, c, e (409, 417)
3 b, d (417)
4 b (412)
5 d (413)
6 e (414–416)
7 d (414–416)
8 e (417)
9 f (418)

PART II

1 a carotid bodies (410)
  b aortic bodies (410)
2 increases; decreases (413)
3 sleep apnea (417)
4 hydrogen-ion concentration (413)
5 hypoxic hypoxia (418)
6 hypoxic hypoxia (417)

13
REGULATION OF WATER AND ELECTROLYTE BALANCE

Module I • Basic principles of renal physiology
Module II • Regulation of sodium and water balance
Module III • Regulation of potassium, calcium, and hydrogen-ion concentrations

Module I • Basic principles of renal physiology

OBJECTIVES

Upon completion of this module, the student will be able to:

1 Define *internal exchanges* and differentiate this from total body input/output.
2 Describe water balance by listing the intakes and outputs.
3 State the major function of the kidney, using the balance concept.
4 State the other general functions of the kidney besides its role in the regulation of the internal environment.
5 Given a diagram of the *nephron* and associated blood vessels, label on the diagram the following items: *glomerulus, Bowman's capsule, proximal tubule, loop of Henle, distal tubule, collecting duct, afferent arteriole, efferent arteriole,* and *peritubular capillaries*; also indicate (using arrows) the direction of blood and glomerular filtrate flow.
6 Given a diagram of a section of the kidney, label the following items: *cortex, medulla, renal pelvis, ureter, bladder,* and *urethra*, and label the direction of glomerular filtrate flow (using arrows).
7 List, define, and locate within the nephron the following basic operations of the

nephron (in any order): *glomerular filtration, tubular secretion,* and *tubular reabsorption.*

8 Define *excretion* and contrast with secretion.

9 Describe the role of *micropuncture* studies in determining the composition of fluid in the renal tubules.

10 State the forces that favor and oppose glomerular filtration.

11 Define *glomerular filtration rate (GFR)* and *filtered load.*

12 State the approximate magnitude of GFR, renal plasma flow, renal blood flow, cardiac output, and total blood volume for a "standard" person.

13 Give the approximate amount of fluid filtered and reabsorbed by the kidneys and excreted as urine per day.

14 Identify active and/or passive processes as part of tubular reabsorption; explain how to prove that a substance has been reabsorbed.

15 Define *maximal tubular capacity (Tm).*

16 State how plasma composition can be regulated by regulating renal absorption and secretion.

17 Explain how to prove that a substance has been secreted.

18 Describe the metabolic functions of the renal tubules.

19 Describe the muscle actions of the bladder and sphincters during *micturition.*

20 Describe the neural control of micturition.

21 Contrast the neural control of micturition in an infant with that in an adult.

READING ASSIGNMENT

Chap. 13, pp. 421–433.

EXERCISES

PART I

424–425 Directions: Answer the following questions in the space provided.

1 Match the forces given in Column A with the pressures (mmHg) given in Column B. For whatever pressures you select for the osmotic gradient, hydrostatic pressure, and glomerular capillary blood pressure, calculate the net filtration pressure.

Column A	Column B
_______ osmotic pressure	a 10
_______ fluid pressure in Bowman's capsule	b 15
	c 30
_______ glomerular capillary blood pressure	d 45
_______ net filtration pressure	e 55
	f 90

2 Label Figs. W-10 and W-11 as indicated. 428

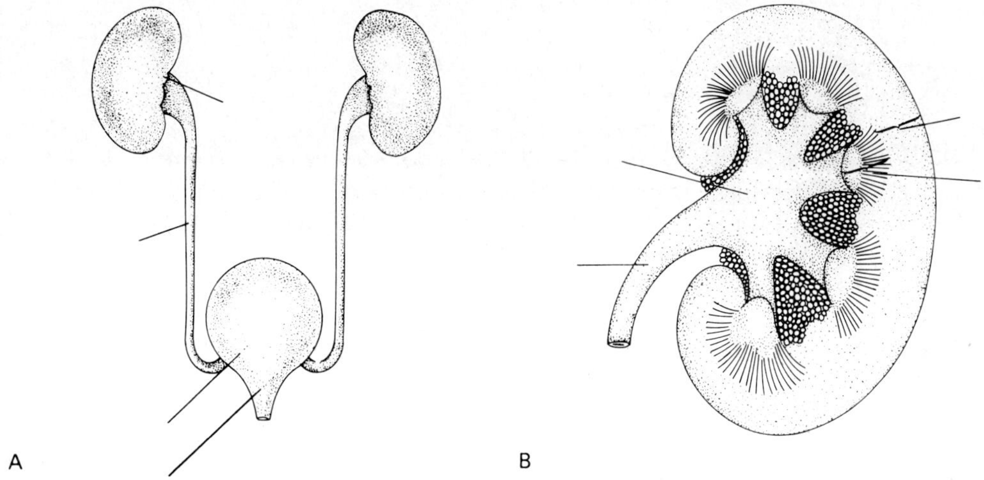

Fig. W-10: Urinary system.

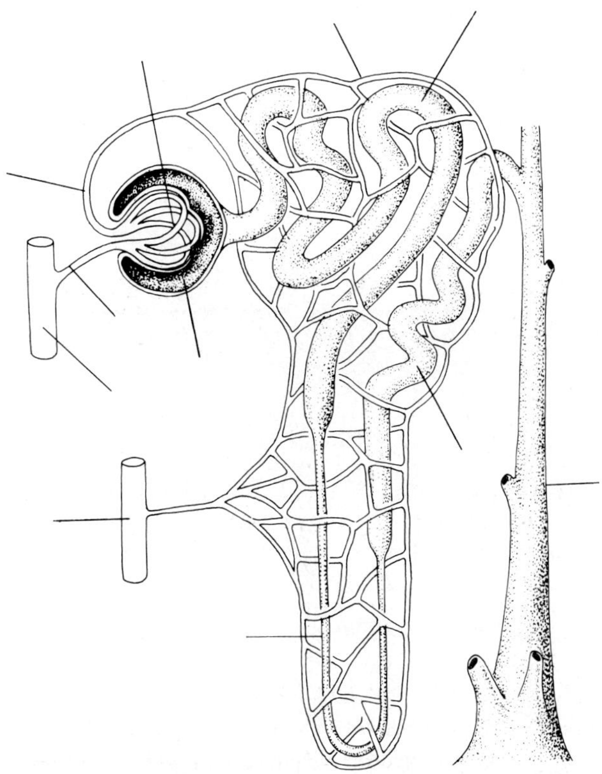

Fig. W-11: Basic structure of a nephron and blood supply.

427 3 Describe how the micropuncture method can be used to determine the composition of the glomerular filtrate.

431 4 Why is glucose excreted in the urine in patients with untreated diabetes mellitus?

425, 432 5 State the four general renal processes responsible for determining the final composition of urine.

433 6 Contrast the neural and muscular control of micturition in the infant with that in the child or adult.

SELF-TEST

PART I

Directions: Answer the following questions in the space provided.

1 Label the following items on Fig. W-12.
- a bladder
- b renal pelvis (on each diagram)
- c direction of urine flow (on each diagram)
- d medullar
- e cortex
- f ureter
- g urethra

2 Label the following items on Fig. W-13.
- a glomerulus
- b Bowman's capsule
- c proximal tubule
- d loop of Henle
- e distal tubule
- f collecting duct
- g afferent arteriole
- h efferent arteriole
- i direction of blood and urine flow (use arrows to indicate)
- j vein
- k artery
- l peritubular capillaries

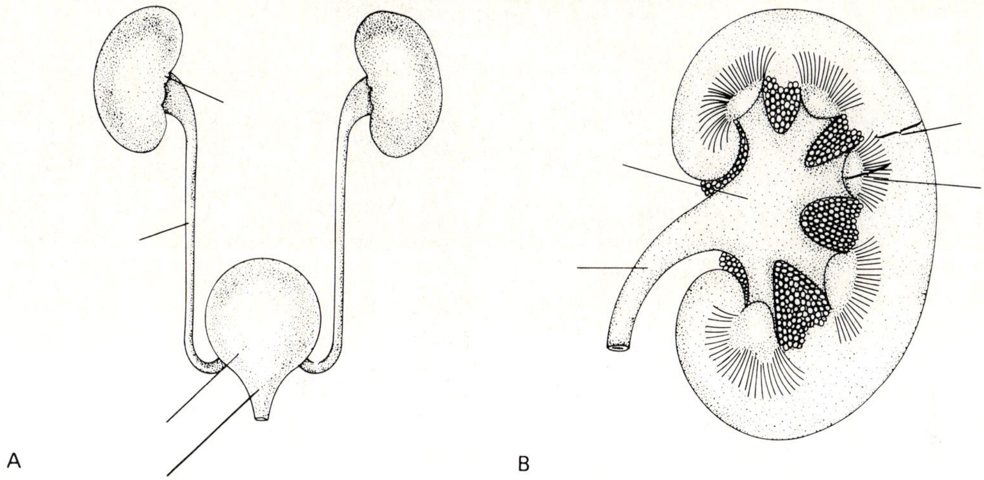

Fig. W-12

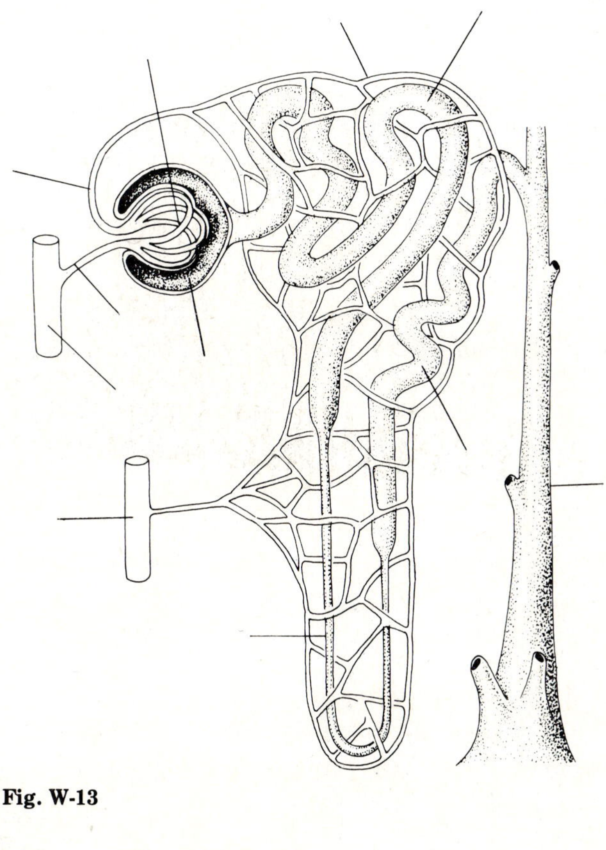

Fig. W-13

PART II

Directions: Circle the correct answer(s).

1 A patient has just had a urinalysis that indicates glucose in the urine. The causes for this could be
  a diabetes mellitus.
  b too little glucose in the plasma.
  c the maximal tubular capacity for glucose has been exceeded.
  d faulty reabsorption of glucose.
  e plasma glucose levels approximately double the normal value.

2 The amount of fluid filtered from the plasma into Bowman's capsule per day is approximately
  a 1–2 L. b 180 L. c 1800 L. d 900 L.

3 Approximately how much fluid is reabsorbed into the peritubular capillaries each day?
  a 99 percent b 10 percent c 50 percent d 1 percent

4 A substance is considered to undergo net secretion by the kidney tubules if its
  a amount in urine is greater than the amount filtered.
  b amount in urine is less than the amount filtered.
  c amount in urine is less than that in plasma.
  d amount in urine is equal to that in plasma.

5 The glomerular filtrate (fluid) in Bowman's capsule
  a has a hydrostatic pressure equal to atmospheric pressure.
  b contains amounts of protein approximately equal to those in plasma.
  c contains all the ions present in plasma in virtually the same concentration as in plasma.
  d contains glucose in essentially the same concentration as in the plasma water that was filtered.

6 Glomerular filtration rate
  a would be expected to decrease in a person who suddenly became hypotensive.
  b would be expected to decrease in a person who suddenly lost a large amount of blood.
  c would be expected to decrease in a person with a partial obstruction of a ureter.
  d would be expected to decrease in response to a large increase in plasma protein concentration.

7 Micturition in infants is initiated by
  a relaxation of skeletal muscles in the pelvic diaphragm.
  b increased sympathetic activity to the bladder.
  c increased parasympathetic activity to the bladder.
  d relaxation of the external urethral sphincter.

Module II • Regulation of sodium and water balance

OBJECTIVES

Upon completion of this module, the student will be able to:

1 Summarize the tubular mechanisms for handling sodium, chloride, and water by the kidney
2 Describe the role of *antidiuretic hormone* in water reabsorption.
3 State the two processes that ultimately define the amount of sodium excreted.
4 State the three reflex pathways by which changes in total body sodium balance lead to changes in GFR and sodium reabsorption.
5 Describe the neural reflex pathway by which GFR is regulated (see Fig. 13–11, p. 437).
6 Describe the role of *aldosterone* in sodium balance.
7 Describe the relation between *renin, angiotensin*, and *aldosterone* (See Fig. 13–12, p. 438).
8 Describe the reflex pathway by which tubular sodium reabsorption is regulated (see Fig. 13–13, p. 439).
9 Describe *natriuretic hormone* and state its role in sodium handling by the kidney.
10 Define *diuretic* and explain its use in treating heart disease.
11 Describe the reflex pathway by which water excretion is altered in response to changes in extracellular volume (see Figs. 13–14 and 13–15, pp. 440–441).
12 Describe how the *countercurrent system* produces a hyperosmotic interstitium in the renal medulla; state how hypotonic or hypertonic urine is formed.
13 Define *osmoreceptors*.
14 Describe the reflex pathway by which water excretion is altered in response to changes in plasma osmolarity (see Fig. 13–18, p. 445).
15 State the primary defect in *diabetes insipidus*.
16 Describe the reflexes contributing to the subjective sensation of thirst (see Fig. 13–20, p. 446).
17 Describe salt appetite.

READING ASSIGNMENT

Chap. 13, pp. 433–446.

EXERCISES

PART I

Directions: In each of the following items, fill in the blank following each phrase to

indicate the change in direction (increases, decreases, or no change) of excretion of Na, Cl, and H_2O under the conditions described. The first part of question 1 is given as an
435–436 example. Fig. 13-9 in the text will be particularly helpful in completing this exercise.

1 When the GFR is normal and reabsorption of Na increases,

a Na excretion ____decreases____

b Cl excretion ________________

c H_2O excretion ________________

2 When the GFR increases and Na reabsorption remains the same,

a Na excretion ________________

b Cl excretion ________________

c H_2O excretion ________________

3 When GFR increases and Na reabsorption decreases,

a Na excretion ________________

b Cl excretion ________________

c H_2O excretion ________________

4 When GFR is normal and Na reabsorption decreases,

a Na excretion ________________

b Cl excretion ________________

c H_2O excretion ________________

PART II

Directions: Answer the following questions in the space provided.

1 For the following variables indicate the direction of change (increase ↑ or decrease
437–441 ↓) that follows salt and water loss due to diarrhea.

a plasma volume
b GFR
c filtered Na
d plasma ADH
e collecting-duct permeability
f urine volume
g aldosterone secretion
h renin secretion
i cardiac output
j Na excreted
k tubular Na reabsorption

2 Show increase or decrease by completing the arrow to the left of each substance. Refer to Fig. 13-13, p. 439, to check your answers. 438

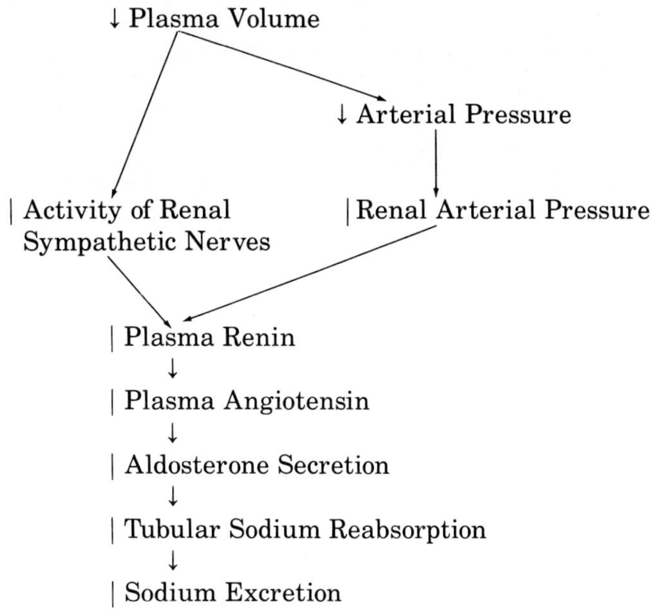

3 Diagram the loop of Henle and an associated collecting duct. Assuming a normal plasma sodium concentration of 300 milliosmol/L and a maximum sodium concentration of 1400 milliosmol/L, write in the existing concentration gradients and the direction of sodium and water movements. See Fig. 13-17, p. 444, to check your answers. 444

4 Describe why urine volume is high, but concentration is low, when a person is secreting very small amounts of ADH. 442

____

____

____

5 Contrast the changes in aldosterone and natriuretic hormone following an evening of beer and pretzels. 436–439

____

____

____

SELF-TEST

PART I

Directions: Complete the following items in the space provided.

1 The reabsorption of sodium is by (a) diffusion or (b) an active process. (Choose one.)

______

2 The reabsorption of water is by (a) diffusion or (b) an active process. (Choose one.)

______

3 The amount of sodium excreted = sodium ______________________________ − sodium ______________________________.

4 In patients whose adrenal glands are removed, large amounts of sodium are excreted in their urine because ______________________________ ______________________________.

5 The hormone that inhibits the reabsorption of sodium is ______________________________.

6 The type of receptor that controls ADH secretion by sensing atrial pressure is known as ______________________________.

7 If the GFR increases and sodium reabsorption decreases, sodium excretion ______________________________.

8 If the GFR decreases and the reabsorption of sodium increases, sodium excretion ______________________________.

9 If GFR increases and sodium reabsorption decreases, water excretion ______________________________.

10 Active sodium transport does not occur in which segment of the loop of Henle?

____

PART II

Directions: Circle the correct answer(s).

1 Complete inhibition of active sodium reabsorption would cause an increase in the excretion of which of the following substances?
   a water   b chloride   c glucose   d red blood cells
2 Which of the following are true of antidiuretic hormone (ADH)?
   a It increases the water permeability of the collecting ducts and the distal tubules.
   b When large amounts are present, the urine excreted has a high osmolarity.
   c Its absence would cause dehydration through excretion of large volumes of urine.
   d It enables proper functioning of the countercurrent multiplier system because it has no direct effect on sodium reabsorption, only on water reabsorption.
3 Which of the following factors *directly* affect GFR?
   a plasma sodium concentration

b plasma calcium concentration
c glomerular capillary blood pressure
d Bowman's capsule hydrostatic pressure
e osmotic pressure due to plasma protein concentration

4 Which of the following correctly describe the reflex pathway relating extracellular volume and water excretion?
a ADH is produced by a group of hypothalamic neurons with axons terminating in the posterior pituitary, from which ADH is released into the blood.
b Vascular baroreceptors, particularly in the left atrium, send information to the hypothalamic neurons involved in ADH secretion.
c The atrial baroreceptors are stimulated by increased atrial blood pressure and in turn send impulses via ascending pathways to the hypothalamus to stimulate ADH-producing cells.
d Decreased atrial pressure causes less firing by the baroreceptors and inhibition of ADH synthesis and release.

5 Which of the following are stimuli that promote thirst?
a drinking ocean salt water
b lower extracellular volume
c higher extracellular volume
d higher plasma osmolarity
e dryness of throat and mouth

6 Which of the following accurately describe the countercurrent-system operation in the kidney?
a Active sodium chloride transport occurs in the descending limb of the loop of Henle.
b The countercurrent system could not operate very long without active sodium chloride transport.
c The highest concentration of sodium chloride is at the tip of the loop of Henle.
d The final urine sodium chloride concentration can never be greater than that at the tip of the loop of Henle.
e If no water diffuses out of the collecting ducts, the urine will be hypotonic.
f The fluid in the descending limb of Henle is always hypoosmotic relative to that of the ascending limb.
g The basic function of the loop countercurrent multiplier system is to concentrate the medullary interstitium.
h Maximum sodium chloride concentration is a function of the length of the loop of Henle and the strength of the sodium pump.
i A person with diabetes insipidus would excrete concentrated urine.
j Final urine concentration occurs in the collecting ducts.
k Hypertonic urine results from low levels of ADH.
l Hypertonic urine is possible because ADH allows water to pass out of the collecting tubules until equilibrium with the medullary interstitium is attained.

7 Inputs that may increase renin release include:
a increased plasma volume.
b decreased activity of renal sympathetic nerves.
c decreased renal arterial blood pressure.
d increased plasma levels of aldosterone.

Module III • Regulation of potassium, calcium, and hydrogen-ion concentrations

OBJECTIVES

Upon completion of this module, the student will be able to:

1 Describe the renal and hormonal control of extracellular potassium ion concentration.
2 Contrast the effects of aldosterone on renal handling of sodium and potassium.
3 List the three effector sites for calcium homeostasis.
4 Identify the mechanisms controlling extracellular calcium concentration by identifying the controlling hormones and the tissues from which they originate, the effects of these hormones, and the substances stimulating the hormone secretion.
5 Describe the role of vitamin D in calcium regulation.
6 Contrast strong acids with weak acids.
7 Describe buffering and buffer systems.
8 List the major buffers in the body.
9 List the major sources of hydrogen ions within the body.
10 Describe the role of bicarbonate-CO_2 as a buffer.
11 State the roles of the kidneys and lungs in hydrogen-ion regulation.
12 State the role of NH_3 and HPO_4^{2-} urinary buffers.
13 Define and describe the two forms of *acidosis* and *alkalosis*.
14 Describe the compensatory changes in metabolic acidosis and alkalosis.
15 Define *uremia*.
16 List the symptoms to expect in patients with advanced renal disease.
17 Describe the artificial kidney.

READING ASSIGNMENT

Chap. 13, pp. 447–458.

EXERCISES

Directions: Answer the following questions in the space provided.

447–448 1 What are the two most important factors controlling potassium plasma concentrations?

____

____

____

2 List three effector sites involved in the regulation of extracellular calcium concentration. **449**

____

____

____

3 Describe four effects of parathyroid hormone on calcium regulation. **450**

____

____

____

____

____

4 Complete the arrows to show an increase or a decrease in the components of the pathway shown. See Fig. 13-22, p. 449, to check your answers.

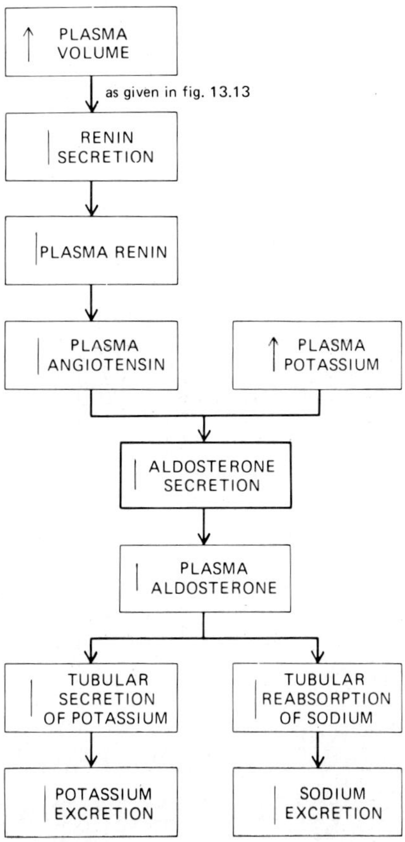

Fig. W-14

5 Complete the arrows to show an increase or a decrease in the components of the pathway shown. See Fig. 13-24, p. 451, to check your answers.

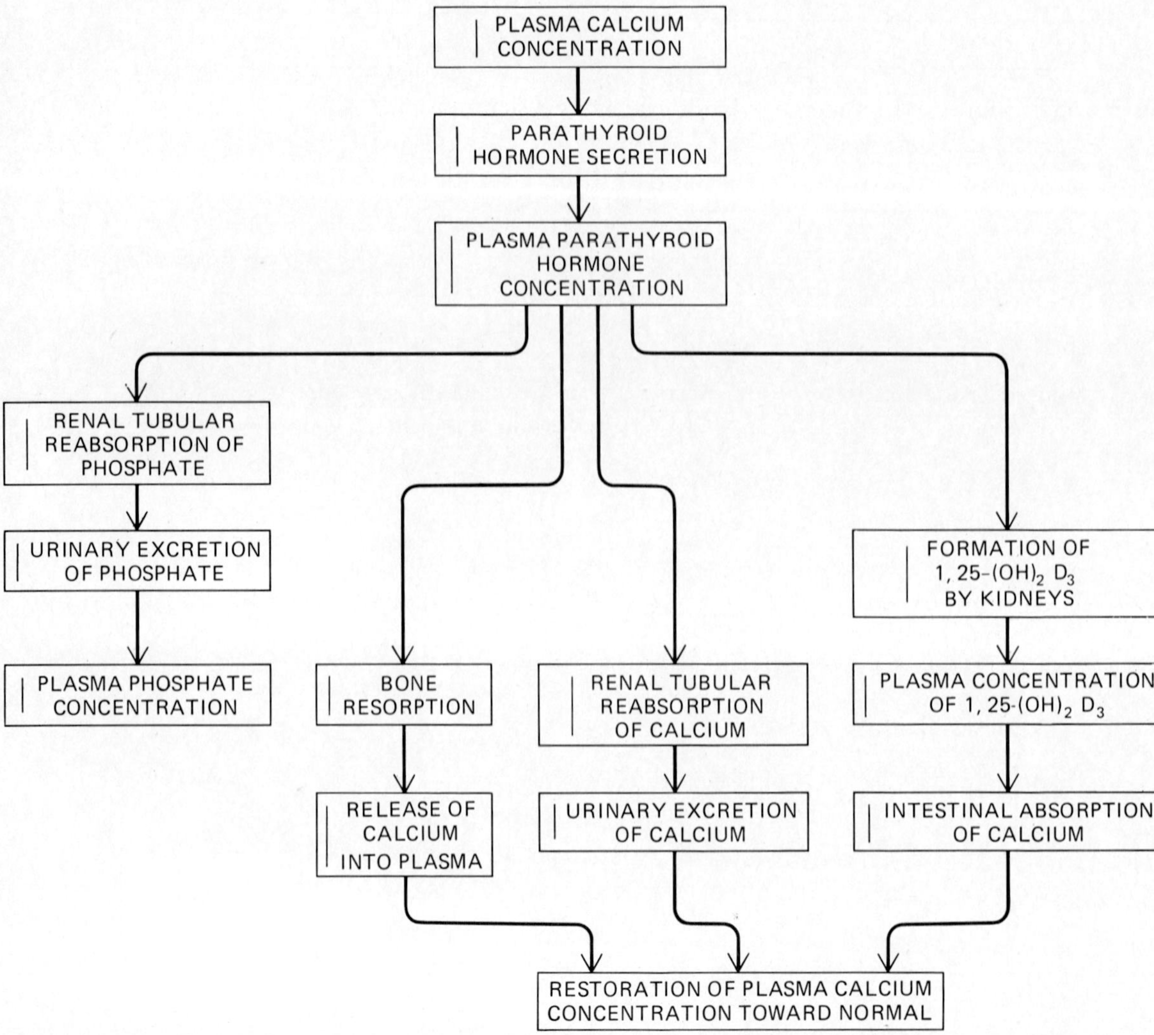

Fig. W-15: Reflexes by which a reduction in plasma calcium concentration is restored toward normal via the actions of parathyroid hormone and vitamin D.

452 6 Explain the difference between a strong and a weak acid.

7 List the major sources of hydrogen ions in the body. 454

____

____

____

8 Discuss the relationship between HCO_{3^-}, H^+, and CO_2 and describe how this system acts as a buffer. 455–456

____

____

____

9 Describe how the lungs participate in acid-base balance. 455

____

____

____

10 Identify the two major hyrogen-ion buffers found in urine and describe how these buffers work. 456

____

____

____

11 Describe the primary defect in each of the following: 457

a metabolic acidosis ______________________________

b metabolic alkalosis ______________________________

c respiratory acidosis ______________________________

d respiratory alkalosis ______________________________

12 Describe how the artificial kidney works. 458

____

____

____

____

SELF-TEST

PART I

Directions: Complete the following items in the space provided.

1 Changes in potassium excretion by the kidney are due to changes in potassium ____________________ (select one: filtration, reabsorption, secretion).

2 High plasma levels of aldosterone result in (increased, decreased) ____________________ potassium excretion.

3 Both parathyroid hormone and calcitonin secretion are altered directly by ____________________.

4 The major action of 1,25-dihydroxyvitamin D_3 is to stimulate active calcium absorption by the ____________________.

5 The process preventing large changes in hydrogen-ion concentration when hydrogen-ion is added to or removed from solution is called ____________________.

6 The three major sources of hydrogen ion in the body are ____________________, ____________________, and ____________________.

7 Virtually all the hydrogen ion excreted in the urine enters the tubules by tubular ____________________.

8 A person hyperventilates. This leads to respiratory (acidosis, alkalosis) ____________________.

9 Vomiting can lead to what type of disorder in hydrogen-ion concentration? ____________________.

10 A person's kidneys are nonfunctioning. This leads to a condition called ____________________.

PART II

Directions: Circle the correct answer(s).

1 In hydrogen-ion regulation in the kidney,
  a reabsorption is the primary regulatory mechanism.
  b secretion is the primary regulatory mechanism.
  c both secretion and reabsorption are regulatory processes.
  d the site of regulation is Bowman's capsule.
  e the site of regulation is the urethra.

2 During hydrogen-ion buffering in the kidney,
  a NH_3 combines with H^+ to become NH_4^+.
  b HPO_4^{2-} combines with H^+ to become H_2PO_{4-}.

c decreased hydrogen-ion concentration results in increased NH_3 excretion in the form of NH_4^+.
d the amount of ammonia that remains in the tubular lumen depends on the rate of hydrogen-ion secretion.

3 Which of the following are true of renal regulation of plasma potassium concentration?
a As in the case for sodium, potassium is completely filterable at the glomerulus.
b Potassium can be reabsorbed but not secreted by the tubules.
c Potassium is not filterable at the glomerulus but is secreted by the renal tubules.
d Reabsorption is not a controlling factor in potassium homeostasis.
e Potassium excretory changes are primarily due to changes in secretion.
f Normal GFR changes do not measurably alter the control of potassium secretion.
g Increases in the plasma concentration of the hormone aldosterone reduce tubular potassium secretion.
h An important control factor is tubule cellular potassium concentration.

4 High calcium levels in the plasma promote which of the following?
a increased parathyroid secretion
b decreased parathryoid secretion
c increased calcitonin secretion
d decreased calcitonin secretion

5 Which are major sources of hydrogen ion in the body?
a bile salts
b hormones
c inorganic acids such as phosphoric and sulfuric acids
d carbonic acid
e organic acids from metabolic reactions

6 Which of the following describe the buffer role of bicarbonate in the equation

$$H^+ + HCO_3^- \underset{2}{\overset{1}{\rightleftharpoons}} H_2CO_3 \underset{4}{\overset{3}{\rightleftharpoons}} H_2O + CO_2$$

a Increased hydrogen ion prompts reaction 1.
b Decreased hydrogen ion prompts reactions 2 and 4.
c All four reactions occur simultaneously in the body.
d Reaction 3 occurs mostly in peripheral tissues.

7 Metabolic acidosis
a can result from vomiting.
b is compensated for by increased ventilation.
c can result from excess production of ketone bodies.
d results in increased amounts of excretion of NH_4^+.

8 Metabolic alkalosis
a can result from excess production of lactic acid.
b can result from fasting.
c can result from vomiting.
d is compensated for by increased ventilation.

9 Respiratory acidosis
  a results from a failure of the lungs to eliminate CO_2 as fast as it is produced.
  b results from ingestion of antacids.
  c results in an elevated arterial CO_2 and H^+.
  d can be caused by fasting.

10 The artificial kidney
  a might be used for a patient with uremia.
  b exchanges wastes between blood and the bath fluid by active transport.
  c exchanges wastes between blood and the bath fluid by bulk-flow.
  d relies on tubing that is permeable only to toxic substances.

Answers

CHAPTER 13 • MODULE I

PART I

1 Check Fig. 13-1, p. 424, for correct labeling
2 Check Figs. 13-2 and 13-3, pp. 425–426, for correct labeling

PART II

1 a, c, d (431)
2 b (429)
3 a (429)
4 a (429)
5 c, d (427–428)
6 a, b, c, d (428–429)
7 c (433)

CHAPTER 13 • MODULE II

PART I

1 b (434)
2 a (434)
3 filtered; reabsorbed (435)
4 absence of aldosterone leads to decreased tubular reabsorption of sodium (437)
5 natriuretic hormone (439)
6 atrial baroreceptor (440)
7 increases (435)
8 decreases (435)
9 increases (435)
10 descending limb (442)

PART II

1 a, b (434–435)
2 a, b, c, d (440–444)
3 c, d, e (plasma sodium concentration, a, does not affect GFR directly) (428)
4 a, b (440)
5 a, b, d, e (446)
6 b, c, d, g, h, j, l (441–444)
7 c (438–439)

CHAPTER 13 • MODULE III

PART I

1 secretion (447)
2 increased (448)
3 plasma calcium concentration (449–452)
4 intestine (450)
5 buffering (453)
6 phosphoric and sulfuric acids, organic acids, carbonic acid (in any order) (454)
7 secretion (456)
8 alkalosis (457)
9 metabolic alkalosis (457)
10 uremia (458)

PART II

1 b (456)
2 a, b, d (456)
3 a, d, e, f, h (447–449)
4 b, c (450–452)
5 c, d, e (454)
6 a, b, c (455–456)
7 b, c, d (456–457)
8 c (457)
9 a, c (457)
10 a (458)

14

DIGESTION AND ABSORPTION OF FOOD

Module I • Overview, and digestion and absorption

OBJECTIVES

Upon completion of this module, the student will be able to:

1 Label a diagram of the anatomy of the gastrointestinal tract (see Fig. 14-1, p. 460) with the following items: parotid salivary glands, pharynx, trachea, esophagus, sublingual and submandibular salivary glands, diaphragm, stomach, pancreas, small intestine, large intestine, gallbladder, liver, appendix, rectum, and anus.
2 Define *digestion, secretion, absorption,* and *motility.*
3 Differentiate between waste leaving the body by the kidneys and lungs and the elimination of *feces.*
4 List three functions of saliva as related to digestion.
5 State the functions of *amylase.*
6 List two functions of hydrochloric acid secretion by the stomach.
7 Define *chyme.*
8 State the function of *pepsin.*
9 List the function of bicarbonate secretion by the exocrine pancreas and liver.
10 State the function of *bile salts* and the *gallbladder.*

11 Label a diagram of a longitudinal section of the wall of the gastrointestinal tract (see Fig. 14-5, p. 466) with the following items: mucosa (including epithelium, lamina propria, and muscularis mucosae), submucosa (including submucus nerve plexus), muscularis externa (including circular smooth muscle, myenteric nerve plexus, and longitudinal smooth muscle), serosa, and ducts from external exocrine glands.

12 Describe the structure of the small intestines, using the terms *duodenum, jejunum, ileum, villi, microvilli,* and *lacteals.*

13 On a diagram of an intestinal villus, label the following structures: microvilli, capillaries, arteries and arterioles, veins and venules, lacteal, and lymph duct.

14 Identify the function of folded mucosa, villi, microvilli, and lacteal.

15 Describe the variable role (depending on the region of the gastrointestinal tract) of tight junctions in the exchange of materials between the lumen of the intestinal tract and the body.

16 Describe the digestion and absorption of carbohydrates, proteins, and fats in the small intestine by listing the principal substrates, enzymes, and sites of activity.

17 Define *emulsification, micelles,* and *chylomicrons.*

18 Describe the absorption of fat-soluble and water-soluble vitamins.

19 Describe the digestion and absorption of nucleic acids.

20 Describe the mechanisms by which water, potassium, calcium, and iron are absorbed from the intestinal tract.

21 Describe the function of *ferritin* and *transferrin* in iron transport and storage.

READING ASSIGNMENT

Chap. 14, pp. 459–475.

EXERCISES

Directions: Answer the following questions in the space provided.

1 On Fig. W-16, a diagram of the anatomy of the gastrointestinal tract, label the
460 following structures:

a parotid salivary gland
b pharynx
c trachea
d esophagus
e sublingual and submandibular salivary glands
f diaphragm
g stomach
h pancreas
i small intestine
j large intestine
k gallbladder
l liver

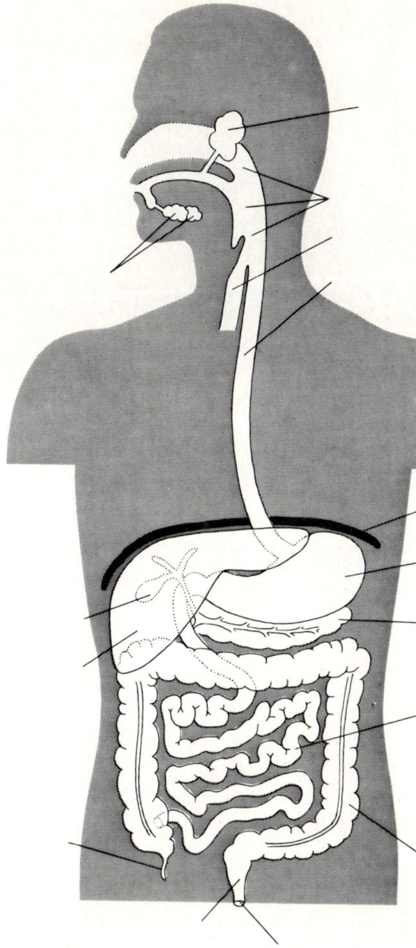

Fig. W-16

m appendix
n rectum
o anus

2 In Fig. W-17 on p. 168 a diagram of a longitudinal section of the gastrointestinal tract, fill in the blank spaces. **466**

3 On Fig. W-18 on p. 168 a diagram of intestinal villi, label the following structures: **470**

a microvilli
b capillaries
c arteries and arterioles
d veins and venules
e lacteal duct
f lymph duct

4 Indicate after each substance whether it is absorbed from the intestinal tract by active-transport mechanisms, by diffusion, or by carrier-mediated transport. **467–475**

a monosaccharides ______________________________

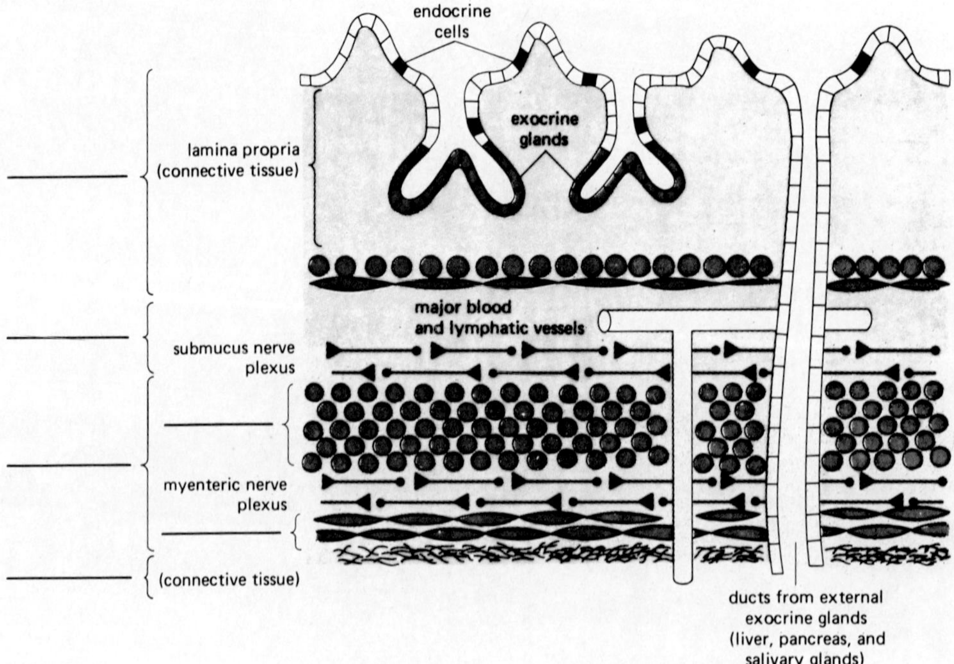

Fig. W-17

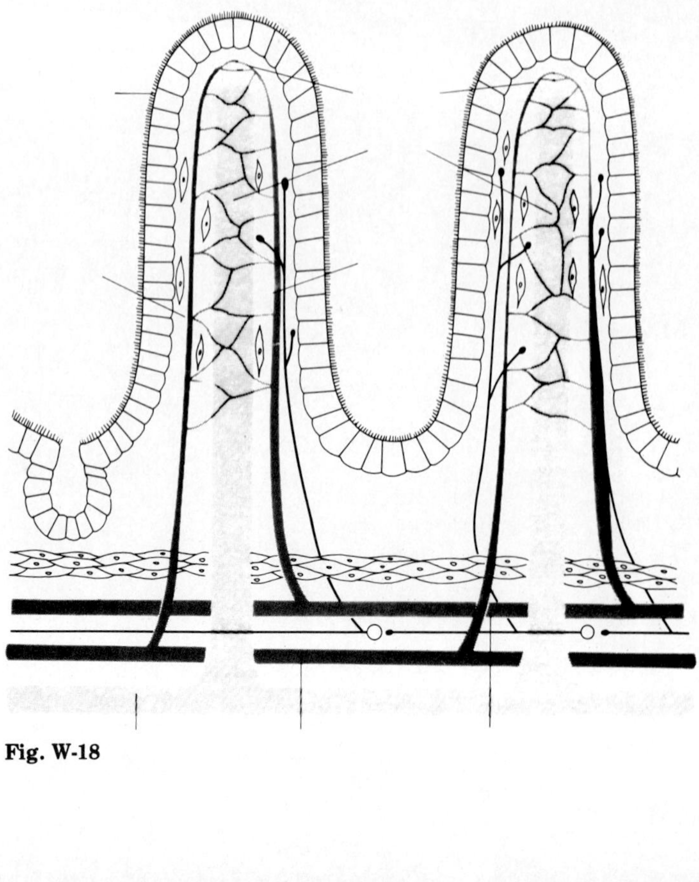

Fig. W-18

b amino acids ______

c free fatty acids ______

d fat-soluble vitamins ______

e water-soluble vitamins ______

f bases from nucleic acids ______

g water ______

h potassium ______

i calcium ______

j iron ______

5 Describe and illustrate the process of fat digestion and absorption including the terms fat droplets, emulsification, bile salts, micelles, lipase, chylomicrons, and lacteals. **470–474; Fig. 14-11, p. 474**

______

______

______

______

______

______

______

______

______

______

SELF-TEST

PART I

Directions: Complete the following items in the space provided.

1 The three pairs of salivary glands are ______, ______, and ______.

2 The partially dissolved food in the stomach is called ______.

3 The segments of the small intestine, beginning from the stomach, are called ______, ______, and ______.

4 Pepsin breaks proteins into ______________________________.

5 The process of breaking up large lipid droplets into smaller lipid droplets is known as ______________________________.

6 Small liquid droplets containing triacylglycerol and small amounts of phospholipid, cholesterol, and fat-soluble vitamins are called ____________________.

7 The most abundant substance in intestinal chyme is ____________________.

8 The absorption of iron varies depending on the ____________________ content of the body.

9 The principal carbohydrate-digesting enzyme in saliva is ________________.

10 The center of each villus has a single blind-ended lymph vessel termed a ______________________________.

PART II

Directions: Circle the correct answer(s).

1 HCl
 a is a weak acid.
 b secretion in the stomach helps to dissolve food particles.
 c secretion in the stomach kills many bacteria.
 d is secreted by glands in the mouth (salivary glands) and in the stomach.

2 Saliva has the following functions:
 a moistens and lubricates food particles.
 b contains the digestive enzyme pepsin.
 c emulsifies fat particles.
 d dissolves some of the molecules in the food.

3 Villi
 a are covered with microvilli.
 b are covered with folded mucosa.
 c increase the surface area of the small intestines.
 d are the sites where most absorption occurs.

4 Which of the following substances are actively transported across the intestinal epithelium?
 a glucose
 b amino acids
 c free fatty acids
 d fat-soluble vitamins
 e nucleotide breakdown products
 f water
 g potassium
 h calcium
 i iron

5 Which of the following statements are correct concerning the transport and storage of iron?
 a Iron is transported into intestinal epithelial cells by diffusion.
 b Inside the intestinal epithelial cells the iron is stored complexed to transferrin.

c Some absorbed iron is released into the plasma and is circulated bound to ferritin.
d In response to a severe hemorrhage the iron bound to ferritin decreases.

Module II • Regulation of the gastrointestinal processes: basic principles

OBJECTIVES

Upon completion of this module, the student will be able to:

1 List the four types of luminal stimuli that trigger gastrointestinal reflexes.
2 Describe the two types of neural reflex pathways linking a stimulus in the gastrointestinal tract to a response.
3 List the three gastrointestinal hormones; describe the major sites of their production, the stimuli inducing their release and inhibition, and the effects on their target cells as given in Table 14-2, p. 478.
4 Identify *bombesin, gastric inhibitory peptide, motilin, somatostatin, vasoactive intestinal peptide,* and *villikinin* as peptides found in the gastrointestinal tract and suspected of being hormones.
5 Define *potentiation* of hormone action.
6 List the three phases of the neural and the hormonal control of the gastrointestinal system and describe the types of stimuli that initiate each phase.

READING ASSIGNMENT

Chap. 14, pp. 475–480.

EXERCISES

Directions: Answer the following questions in the space provided.

1 After each hormone, list the major site of its production, the stimuli for inducing its release, and its effects on various target cells. 478

a gastrin ______________________________

____

____

b secretin ______________________________

____

____

c cholecystokinin ______________________________

____

____

480 2 The luminal stimuli capable of initiating most gastrointestinal reflexes include the following:

a ______________________________

b ______________________________

c ______________________________

d ______________________________

479–480 3 For each of the three phases of gastrointestinal control, list the stimuli responsible for initiating the reflex.

a cephalic phase ______________________________

____

____

b gastric phase ______________________________

____

____

c intestinal phase ______________________________

____

____

SELF-TEST

PART I

Directions: Complete the following items in the space provided.

1 Four types of intraluminal stimuli that induce gastrointestinal reflexes are ______________, ______________, ______________, and ______________.

2 The neural and hormonal control of the gastrointestinal system is divisible into

three phases—____________________, ____________________, and ____________________.

3 The neural reflex pathways controlling gastrointestinal function are categorized into ____________________ reflexes and ____________________ reflexes.

4 The three gastrointestinal hormones are ____________________, ____________________, and ____________________.

5 The presence of a low concentration of a hormone might result in the enhanced secretion of some substance in response to another hormone. This process is known as ____________________.

PART II

Directions: Circle the correct answer(s).

1 Secretin
   a is a hormone produced primarily in the stomach.
   b is released when there is acid in the small intestine.
   c stimulates pancreatic bicarbonate secretion.
   d stimulates gastric secretion.

2 Cholecystokinin
   a is a hormone produced by the liver.
   b is released when there is acid in the stomach.
   c stimulates pancreatic enzyme secretion.
   d stimulates gallbladder contraction.

3 Gastrin
   a is a hormone produced by the antrum of the stomach.
   b is released following ingestion of protein.
   c stimulates acid secretion.
   d stimulates antral contractions.

4 Which of the following are peptides found in the gastrointestinal tract and are suspected of being hormones?
   a somatostatin
   b motilin
   c villikinin
   d pepsinogen
   e bombesin

Module III • Regulation of the gastrointestinal processes: from mouth to anus

Upon completion of this module, the student will be able to:

1 List the major components of saliva.
2 Describe the neural control of salivation.
3 Describe the act of swallowing taking into account the pressures in the pharynx, thoracic esophagus, and stomach, the *upper esophageal sphincter* and the *lower esophageal sphincter, peristaltic waves,* and *secondary peristalsis.*
4 State the physiological reasons for "heartburn" during the last 5 months of pregnancy.
5 List the secretions of the *mucous cells,* the *parietal cells* (*oxyntic cells*), and the *chief cells.*
6 Label the following structures on a diagram of the stomach: *esophagus, fundus, body, antrum, pyloric sphincter,* and *duodenum.*
7 Describe the three major exocrine secretions of the stomach and the cells involved.
8 Describe the cellular processes involved in the secretion of HCl by the parietal cells.
9 Describe the factors controlling HCl secretion by the stomach.
10 Describe the pathways and cells regulating the secretion and activation of pepsinogen in the stomach.
11 Define *receptive relaxation* and *basic electrical rhythm* of the stomach.
12 Describe the factors controlling gastric motility and emptying.
13 List the types of stimuli that can induce vomiting.
14 Describe the act of vomiting.
15 Name the exocrine secretions of the pancreas; state their roles in digestion.
16 Describe the roles of *enterokinase* and *trypsin* on the activation of pancreatic enzymes.
17 Describe the factors controlling pancreatic enzyme secretion.
18 List the six primary ingredients of bile.
19 Identify the sites of formation and storage of bile.
20 Describe the role of the *enterohepatic circulation* in bile-salt recycling.
21 Describe the factors that control bile secretion.
22 Describe the reasons for water movement into the lumen of the small intestine.
23 Describe the secretions of the small intestine.
24 Define *segmentation;* describe its control.
25 Describe the roles of segmentation and peristalsis (*migrating motility complex*) in moving food down the small intestine.
26 Define *gastroileal reflex, ileogastric reflex,* and *intestino-intestinal reflex.*
27 List the six segments of the large intestine.
28 List the substances that are absorbed or secreted by the large intestine.
29 Define *mass movement;* describe its role in the initiation of defecation.
30 Describe the process of defecation.

READING ASSIGNMENT

Chap. 14, pp. 480–500.

EXERCISES

Directions: Answer the following questions in the space provided.

1 On Fig. W-19, a diagram of the stomach, label the following items: **483**

a	esophagus	d	antrum
b	fundus	e	pyloric sphincter
c	body	f	duodenum

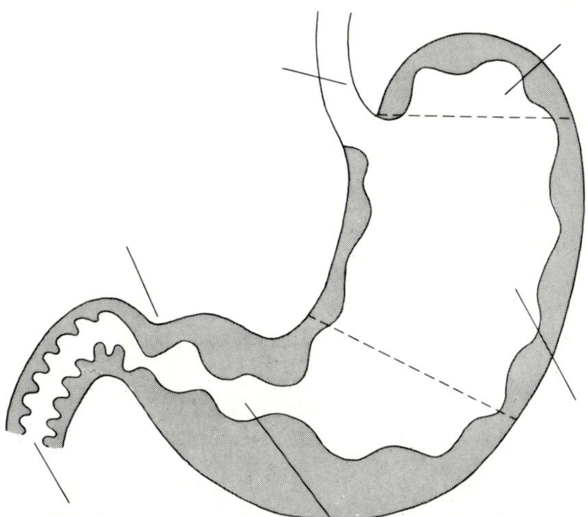

Fig. W-19

2 Describe why a person can swallow while upside down. **482**

3 Why do you suppose that before a meal the pH of the stomach contents is lower (greater hydrogen-ion concentration) than shortly after ingestion when acid secretion is increased? **486**

4 Why is it significant that pepsin is secreted in an inactive form? **486**

5 Describe the process by which acid secretion by the stomach is neutralized by pancreatic secretions. How does this contribute to the overall acid-base balance of
491 the body?

6 Why is it that during a meal as much as 8 g of bile salts can be emptied into the
494 duodenum when the total body content of bile salts may be only approximately 4 g?

7 Why should there be a net influx of water across the wall of the small intestine
495 from the blood into the lumen following a meal?

496–497 8 How does segmentation propel food down the small intestine?

499 9 Describe the stimuli for the initiation and the actual process of defecation.

SELF-TEST

PART I

Directions: Complete the following items in the space provided.

1 Compared to atmospheric pressure, the pressures in the (a) pharynx, (b) thoracic esophagus, and (c) stomach are, respectively, ________, ________, and ________.

2 Hydrochloric acid is secreted by ______________________ cells.

3 The rhythmicity in the longitudinal muscles of the stomach (approximately 3/min) is called ______________________.

4 The ______________________ sphincter prevents food from leaving the stomach and entering the duodenum.

5 The enzyme ______________________ splits off a peptide from pancreatic trypsinogen, forming the active enzyme ______________________, which activates the other proteolytic enzyme precursors from the pancreas.

6 From the standpoint of gastrointestinal function, the ______________________ are the most important components of bile.

7 The recycling of bile salts from the intestine to the liver and back to the intestine is known as the ______________________.

8 Contractile activity in the ileum increases during periods of gastric emptying. This is called the ______________________.

9 The increased motility in the large intestine, causing propulsion of fecal material up to three-fourths of the length of the colon in a few seconds, is called ______________________.

10 In children and adults, voluntary control exists over the ______________________ anal spincter.

PART II

Directions: Circle the correct answer(s).

1 During swallowing,
  a the swallowing center inhibits respiration.
  b the glottis opens while food is in the pharynx.
  c peristaltic waves move the food from the esophagus to the stomach.
  d the lower esophageal sphincter is relaxed until the bolus of food enters the stomach.

2 Pepsinogen
  a is secreted by chief cells.
  b is converted to its active form, pepsin, by the high pH (low acidity) in the stomach.
  c is converted to its active form, pepsin, by the presence of pepsin in the stomach (a positive-feedback process).
  d in its active form helps to digest carbohydrates.

3 HCl
  a secretion is inhibited by the enzyme carbonic anhydrase.
  b secretion increases as signals from the vagus nerve increase.
  c secretion increases with distension of the stomach.

d secretion increases with distension of the duodenum.
e secretion increases with high acidity in the duodenum.

4 Gastric secretions
a consist primarily of a basic solution (pH greater than 7.0) before food reaches the stomach.
b of HCl are increased by increased levels of gastrin.
c of gastrin are stimulated by the presence of peptides in the stomach.
d are inhibited when there is fat in the duodenum.
e are inhibited by hypertonic solutions in the duodenum.

5 Gastric motility
a increases with distension of the stomach.
b increases with distension of the duodenum.
c increases with the presence of fat in the duodenum.
d increases with elevated plasma concentrations of gastrin.

6 Vomiting can be triggered by which of the following stimuli?
a excessive distension of the stomach or small intestine.
b increased pressure within the head.
c intense pain.
d chemical stimuli in the stomach.

7 Bicarbonate secretion by the pancreas
a results in neutralization of the intestinal acid secretions by the stomach.
b results in neutralization of blood bicarbonate secretion by the stomach.
c increases in response to the release of the hormone CCK.
d increases in response to the presence of fat in the duodenum.

8 Bile
a is produced in the pancreas and stored in the gallbladder.
b salts are recycled in a process known as the hepatocyte rotation.
c salt secretion is stimulated by high plasma concentrations of bile salts.
d release from the gallbladder is stimulated by high plasma concentrations of gastrin.

9 Which of the following statements are true concerning small-intestine motility?
a Segmentation rate in the duodenum is more rapid than in the ileum.
b The magnitude of segmentation is dependent entirely on nerve activity and is independent of hormonal levels.
c Peristalsis does not occur in the small intestine, but only in the esophagus and stomach.
d Large distensions of the intestine result in increased motor activity (the intestino-intestinal reflex).

10 The process of defecation
a is often initiated by distension of the walls of the rectum.
b is generally assisted by a deep inspiration followed by closure of the glottis.
c often results in a sharp fall in intraabdominal pressure, as the abdominal and chest muscles contract.
d can often be consciously prevented by descending pathways from the brain to the internal anal sphincter.

Module IV • Pathophysiology of the gastrointestinal tract

OBJECTIVES

Upon completion of this module, the student will be able to:

1 List the factors that prevent the stomach from self-digestion.
2 Define *ulcers;* list possible factors leading to ulceration.
3 Define *gallstones;* list possible factors leading to gallstone production.
4 Describe the effects of gallstones lodging in the common bile duct.
5 Define and describe the effects of *lactose intolerance.*
6 Describe the symptoms (and the causes) of *constipation.*
7 List possible factors contributing to constipation.
8 Describe how laxatives might work to promote defecation.
9 Define *diarrhea;* list possible factors leading to diarrhea.
10 Describe the harmful effects of severe diarrhea.

READING ASSIGNMENT

Chap. 14, pp. 500–503.

EXERCISES

Directions: After each gastrointestinal malfunction, define the term and list factors (or the factor) that might result in the malfunction.

1 ulcers ____________________

____

____________________ **500**

2 gallstones ____________________

____

____________________ **501**

3 lactose intolerance ____________________

____

____________________ **500–501**

4 constipation ____________________

____

502 ______________________________

5 diarrhea ______________________________

____

502–503 ______________________________

SELF-TEST

Directions: Circle the correct answer(s).

1 Factors that protect the stomach from self-digestion are
  a the mucosal surface, which is slightly acidic.
  b the presence of proteins in mucus lining the mucosal surface.
  c the presence of tight junctions between epithelial cells.
  d the rapid replacement of the epithelial cells.
2 A gallstone lodged in the common bile duct can
  a cause pain.
  b increase the digestion of fats in the small intestine.
  c result in diarrhea.
  d lead to jaundice.
3 Which of the following statements are true concerning lactose intolerance?
  a The afflicted person cannot digest starch.
  b The enzyme pepsin is produced in inadequate amounts.
  c The enzyme responsible for digesting lactose often increases in concentration in individuals as they age.
  d The inability to digest lactose can result in gas production, fluid in the large intestine, and diarrhea.
4 The symptoms of constipation can be caused by
  a toxins in the lower intestines.
  b distension of the rectum.
  c eating dietary fiber.
  d ingesting laxatives.

Answers

CHAPTER 14 • MODULE I

PART I

1 parotid, submandibular, sublingual glands (460)
2 chyme (461)
3 duodenum; jejenum; ileum (465)
4 peptides (461)
5 emulsification (471)
6 chylomicrons (473)
7 water (473)
8 iron (475)
9 amylase (461)
10 lacteal (466)

PART II

1 b, c (461)
2 a, d (461)
3 a, c, d (465)
4 a, b, e, h, i (469–475)
5 d (475)

CHAPTER 14 • MODULE II

PART I

1 distension, osmolarity of chyme, acidity, end products of digestion (in any order) (480)
2 cephalic, gastric, intestinal (in any order) (479–480)
3 short, long (in any order) (476)
4 secretin, cholecystokinin (CCK), gastrin (in any order) any order) (477)
5 potentiation (479)

PART II

1 b, c (478)
2 c, d (478)
3 a, b, c, d (478)
4 a, b, c, e (479)

CHAPTER 14 • MODULE III

PART I

1 (a) atmospheric; (b) −5 to −10 mmHg; (c) greater than atmospheric (481)
2 parietal or oxyntic cells (483)
3 basic electrical rhythym (488)
4 pyloric (488)
5 enterokinase; trypsin (492)
6 bile salts (494)
7 enterohepatic circulation (494)
8 gastroileal reflex (497)
9 mass movement (499)
10 external (499)

PART II

1 a, c, d (481–482)
2 a, c (486)
3 b, c (484–485)
4 b, c, d, e (484–486)
5 a, d (489)
6 a, b, c, d (490)
7 a, b, c, d (491–493)
8 c (494–495)
9 a (496–497)
10 a, b (499)

CHAPTER 14 • MODULE IV

1 b, c, d (500)
2 a, c, d (501)
3 d (501–502)
4 b (502)

15
REGULATION OF ORGANIC METABOLISM AND ENERGY BALANCE

Module I • Absorptive and postabsorptive states

OBJECTIVES

Upon completion of this module, the student will be able to:

1. Define and list the three categories of *essential nutrients.*
2. Differentiate between high- and low-quality proteins.
3. Identify the following as characteristics of carbohydrate, fat, and amino acid catabolism: (a) The major fate of both fat and carbohydrate is catabolism to yield energy, whereas amino acids can supply energy only after they are converted to carbohydrate or fat; (b) excess carbohydrate and fat can be stored as such, whereas excess amino acids are not stored as protein but are converted to fat and carbohydrate.
4. Diagram the major inputs and outputs of the protein, carbohydrate, and fat pools (see Fig. 15-1, p. 506, and Fig. 15-2, p. 507).

5 Define *absorptive* and *postabsorptive state.*
6 List the four characteristics of the absorptive state and the three characteristics of the postabsorptive state.
7 Describe the roles played by glucose in the liver in fat synthesis.
8 Describe the fate of most fat synthesized by the liver.
9 State the three major sources of fatty acids found in adipose-tissue triacylglycerol.
10 Contrast the absorptive and postabsorptive states in terms of *anabolism* and *catabolism.*
11 Diagram or list all the major events of the postabsorptive period in terms of blood glucose regulation.
12 List the sources of blood glucose during the postabsorptive state.
13 Define *gluconeogenesis.*
14 Define *glucose sparing* and describe its adaptive significance.
15 Define *ketone bodies.*
16 Identify the changes occurring in brain metabolism during prolonged fasting and the significance of these changes in terms of body functioning.

READING ASSIGNMENT

Chap. 15, pp. 504–513.

EXERCISES

Directions: Answer the following questions in the space provided.

1 a Describe the general fate of ingested glucose during the absorptive state. **508–510**

______

______

______

b Identify the sources of blood glucose during the postabsorptive state. **511**

______

______

______

2 Describe the three major sources of adipose-tissue triacylglycerol. **510**

a ______

______

b ______

c ____

____

507 3 Complete Fig. W-20, a diagram of carbohydrate and fat metabolism, by drawing arrows on the connecting lines to indicate direction of flow.

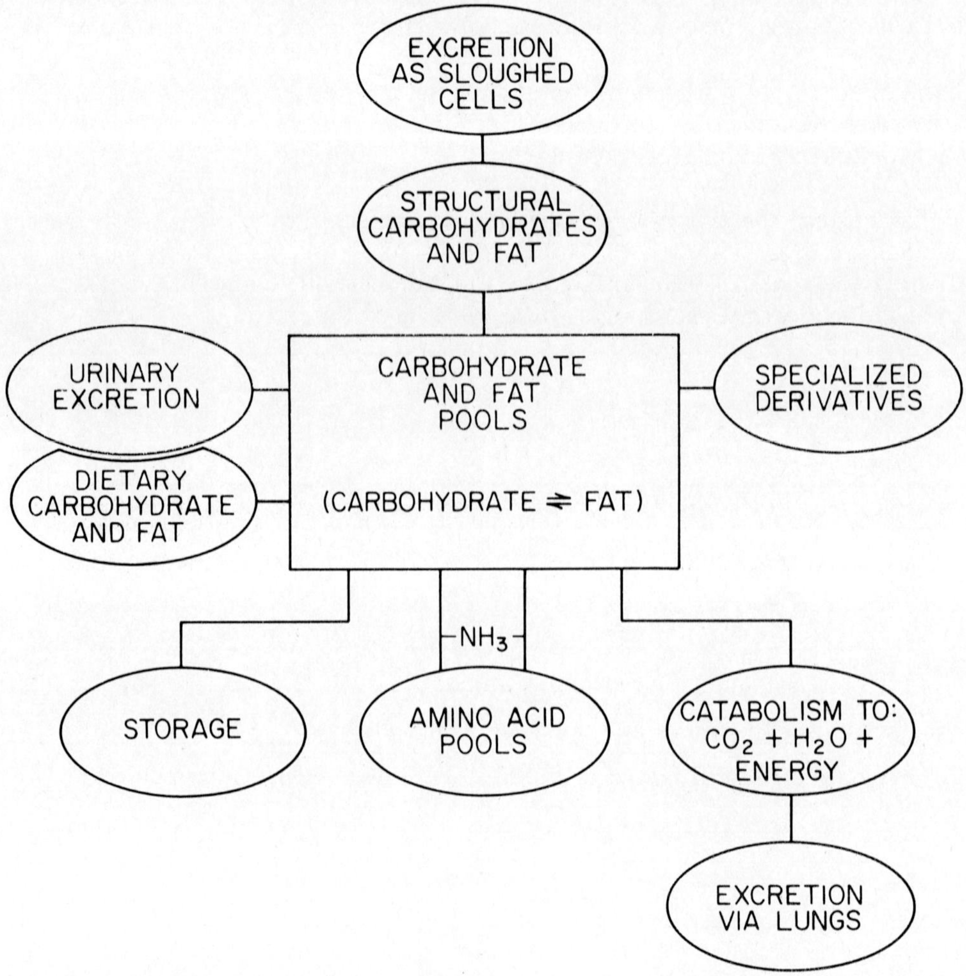

Fig. W-20. Carbohydrate and fat metabolism.

506 4 Complete Fig. W-21, a diagram of protein metabolism, by drawing arrows on the connecting lines to indicate direction of flow.

508, 510 5 Describe the possible metabolic interconversions of ingested amino acids.

____

____

____

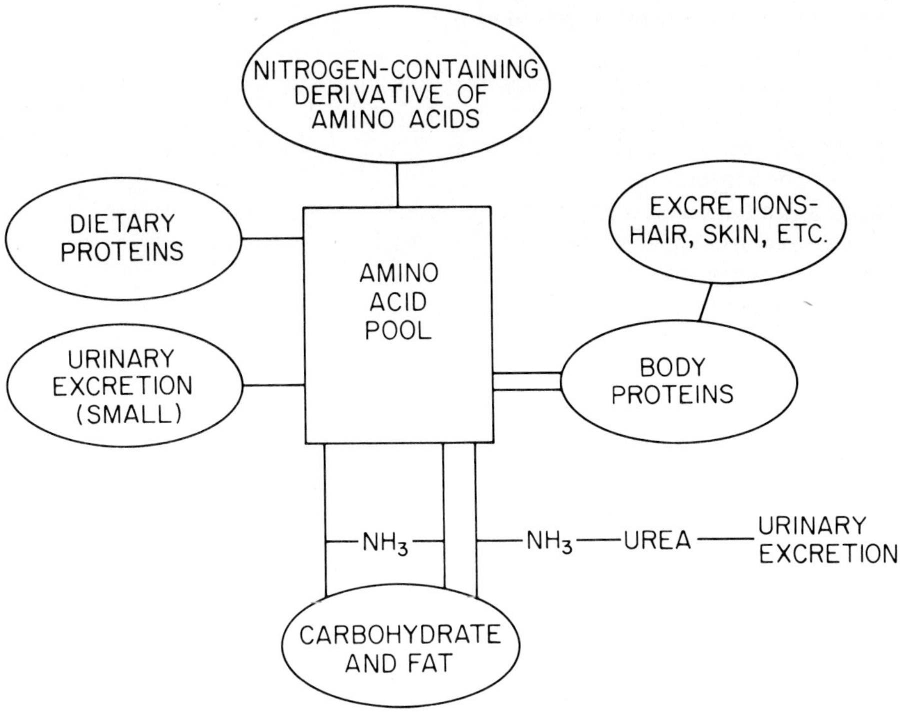

Fig. W-21. Protein metabolism.

6 Describe why during a prolonged fast blood glucose cannot provide all the energy needed by the body. **511**

____

____

____

SELF-TEST

Directions: Circle the correct answer(s).

1 During fasting, blood glucose may be available from
  a glycogen stores in the liver.
  b glycogen stores in muscle.
  c triacylglycerols.
  d muscle protein.
2 During prolonged fasting,
  a body processes alter so as to preserve the plasma glucose level.
  b ketone bodies are formed.

c amino acids are converted to glucose.
d gluconeogenesis takes place.

3 Which of the following occur during the absorptive phase of digestion?
a Glucose provides the major source of energy.
b A large percentage of the amino acids, fats, and carbohydrates are transformed into adipose-tissue fat.
c Many amino acids enter the liver where they are converted to keto acids.
d Glycogen is broken down to glucose in the liver.

4 During the absorptive state
a glycogen is being produced and stored in the liver and muscle.
b most ammonia is being converted to urea in the kidney.
c VLDL are being released from adipose tissue and transported to the liver.
d VLDLs are being produced, and since these lipoproteins are lipid-soluble, they easily diffuse across capillary walls.

5 Which of the following occur during the postabsorptive state?
a Triacylglycerols are catabolized to glycerol and fatty acids.
b Glycogen can supply energy needs for approximately 24 h.
c Proteins provide little source of blood glucose.
d Blood glucose concentration falls rapidly to low levels.

6 To summarize the major metabolic pathways for carbohydrate, fat, and protein:
a excess carbohydrate and fat can be stored as such.
b excess amino acids can supply energy only after they are converted to carbohydrate or fat.
c the major fate of both carbohydrate and fat is catabolism to yield energy.
d excess amino acids are not stored as protein but are converted to carbohydrate and fat.

7 Anabolism exceeds catabolism when
a a person is in the postabsorptive state.
b a person is fasting.
c a person is in the absorptive state.
d a person is on a low calorie, but high protein, diet.

Module II • Endocrine and neural control of absorptive and postabsorptive states

OBJECTIVES

Upon completion of this module, the student will be able to:

1 Identify the cellular sources of the pancreatic hormones *insulin, glucagon, somatostatin,* and *pancreatic polypeptide.*

2 Describe the major categories of effects of insulin on target cells.
3 Describe the transport, anabolic, and catabolic actions of insulin on glycogen synthesis and triacylglycerol storage.
4 State the effects of insulin deficit.
5 Describe the multiple controls of insulin secretion.
6 Describe the metabolic events occurring in a person who has untreated *diabetes mellitus.*
7 Distinguish between *Type 1* (insulin-dependent) and *Type 2* (insulin-independent) diabetes.
8 Describe the renal function and the respiratory compensations of a patient with untreated Type 1 diabetes mellitus.
9 Describe the postulated mechanism by which chronic overeating can lead to Type 2 diabetes.
10 Describe the major effects of glucagon on organic metabolism.
11 Describe the multiple controls of glucagon secretion.
12 State the effects of glucagon deficit and excess.
13 Describe the multiple controls and effects of pancreatic somatostatin.
14 State the effects of epinephrine on (a) secretion of insulin and glucagon and on (b) *glycogenolysis, gluconeogenesis,* and *fat mobilization.*
15 Describe the role of the sympathetic nervous system in the regulation of plasma glucose and fatty acid concentrations.
16 Describe the role of cortisol and growth hormone on organic metabolism and on the metabolic adaptations to fasting and stress.
17 Define *hypoglycemia.*
18 List the fuels used during the early, middle, and late phases of endurance exercise.
19 Describe the hormonal regulation of plasma fuel levels during exercise.
20 Define *low-density lipoproteins, high-density lipoproteins,* and *cholesterol.*
21 List the sources of gain and loss of body cholesterol.
22 Describe the homeostatic control of plasma cholesterol.
23 Describe the relationship between the intake of saturated and unsaturated fats and the plasma cholesterol concentration.
24 Describe the relationship between LDL and HDL and plasma cholesterol.

READING ASSIGNMENT

Chap. 15, pp. 513–529.

EXERCISES

Directions: Answer the following questions in the space provided.

1 Describe the effects that insulin has on membrane transport and on enzyme anabolic and catabolic pathways. **513–514**

____

516 2 List the multiple neural and hormonal controls of insulin secretion.

3 Why might a person with untreated Type I diabetes mellitus have an increased
517 respiratory rate?

4 Explain why weight reduction is thought to often alleviate the symptoms of Type
518 2 diabetes.

5 What is the adaptive value of the secretion of glucagon increasing in response to
520 an elevated plasma amino acid concentration?

6 You are nervous before an examination. Describe the effect of increased sympa-
521–522 thetic neural activation on organic metabolism.

523 7 Contrast cortisol's permissive effect during fasting with its effects during stress.

8 Why do plasma glucagon levels rise and plasma insulin levels fall during periods
525 of exercise when plasma glucose concentration is stable or even elevated?

____

____

9 "Plasma cholesterol levels can simply be controlled by reducing the ingestion of foods high in cholesterol." Defend or refute this statement. 527–529

____

____

____

SELF-TEST

PART I

Directions: Complete the following items in the space provided.

1 Identify the islet of Langerhans' cells that secrete

a glucagon ______________

b somatostatin ______________

c pancreatic polypeptide ______________

d insulin ______________

2 Insulin secretion is directly controlled by the concentration of ______________ and ______________ in the blood flowing through the pancreas.

3 In the untreated Type 1 diabetic, plasma levels of glucose might rise to such a high level that glucose is excreted in the ______________.

4 In Type 2 diabetes, it is postulated that the number of ______________ receptors is decreased in response to a chronically elevated plasma glucose concentration.

5 Indicate whether plasma glucose concentration increases or decreases after administration of each of the following substances.

a insulin ______________

b glucagon ______________

c epinephrine ______________

d cortisol ______________

e growth hormone ______________

6 The technical name for a blood glucose concentration below the normal value is ______________.

7 The major carrier of cholesterol in plasma is ______________________.

8 Ingestion of ______________________ (choose one: saturated or unsaturated) fatty acids tends to raise plasma cholesterol, both by stimulating cholesterol synthesis and by inhibiting cholesterol conversion to ______________________.

PART II

Directions: Circle the correct answer(s).

1 Which of the following are stimulated directly or indirectly by insulin?
   a glucose synthesis
   b glycogen synthesis
   c fat synthesis
   d amino acid transport into cells.

2 In a person with untreated Type 1 diabetes mellitus, lowered insulin concentration results in
   a catabolism of triacylglycerols into fatty acids and ketone bodies.
   b metabolic acidosis.
   c increased respiratory rate.
   d weight gain.

3 Which of the following result in an increase in the secretion of insulin?
   a increased sympathetic neural activity
   b increased parasympathetic neural activity
   c increased plasma amino acid concentration
   d increased plasma glucose concentration

4 Glucagon secretion
   a leads to increased gluconeogenesis.
   b results in increased glycogenolysis.
   c increases during the postabsorptive state.
   d increases in response to an elevation in plasma amino acid concentration.

5 Increased activity of the sympathetic nervous system
   a raises the plasma concentration of epinephrine.
   b results in glycogenolysis.
   c results in increased fat storage.
   d stimulates insulin secretion.

6 A marked increase in the plasma concentration of cortisol results in
   a increased protein synthesis.
   b decreased liver uptake of amino acids.
   c reduced mobilization of adipose tissue fat.
   d increased glucose uptake by most tissues.

7 During short bouts of moderate exercise
   a blood glucose concentration falls rapidly.
   b increased sympathetic activity to the pancreas results in increased secretion of glucagon.
   c glucose uptake by muscles increases.
   d plasma insulin levels tend to rise.

8 Which of the following statements are true concerning the regulation of plasma cholesterol?
   a Plasma cholesterol circulates mainly bound to high-density lipoproteins.
   b Cholesterol is lost via excretion in the urine and catabolism to bile pigments.
   c Doubling of ingested cholesterol will result in an approximate doubling of the plasma cholesterol level.
   d High intake of unsaturated fats stimulates the synthesis of cholesterol from the liver.

Module III • Control of growth

OBJECTIVES

Upon completion of this module, the student will be able to:

1 Define critical period of development, and differentiate among the critical period for brain, total body, and reproductive organs.
2 Differentiate between true growth and a simple gain in weight.
3 Define *osteoblasts* and *epiphyseal plates.*
4 State the relation between an individual's growth capacity and environmental (external) factors.
5 List the five hormones that exert the most important effects on human growth.
6 Describe the metabolic effects of growth hormone on growth in children and in adults.
7 Describe the effects of growth hormone and other factors on the secretion of *somatomedins* and other *insulin-like growth factors.*
8 Describe the burst secretion pattern of growth hormone and the effects of age on the total 24-h secretion of growth hormone.
9 Describe the factors controlling the secretion of growth hormone.
10 Describe the effects of thyroid hormones on growth.
11 Describe the role of insulin in growth.
12 Describe the effect of androgens and estrogens on general body growth.
13 Describe the effects of cortisol on growth.
14 Define, and give an example of, *compensatory growth.*

READING ASSIGNMENT

Chap. 15, pp. 529–533.

EXERCISES

Directions: Answer the following questions in the space provided.

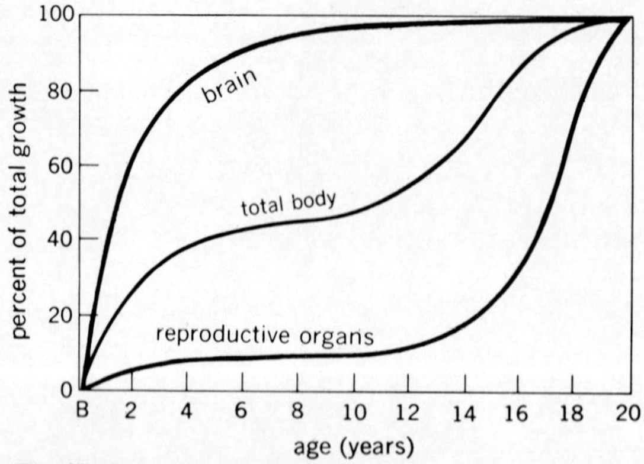

Fig. W-22

529–530 1 Describe what Fig. W-22 tells you about critical periods of growth and the possible results of temporary malnutrition

530–531 2 Describe the multiple effect of growth hormone on growth.

533 3 Why might growth be stunted during an illness?

531 4 A normal amount of thyroid hormone is necessary for normal growth. Will administration of excess thyroid hormone lead to excess growth? What will be its effects?

531 5 Describe the possible effects resulting from deficient thyroid hormone activity during growth.

6 Explain why injection of androgens in small children may result in the premature stoppage of growth. 533

---

7 Contrast normal and compensatory growth. 533

SELF-TEST

Directions: Circle the correct answer(s).

1 Hormone(s) that act to stop bone growth by inducing conversion of the epiphyseal plate to bone is (are)
   a growth hormone. b thyroid hormones. c androgens. d glucagon.
2 Acromegaly results from an increase in hormone(s) after loss of the actively growing cartilage in long bones. The hormone(s) responsible is (are)
   a growth hormone. b thyroid hormones. c androgens. d estrogen.
3 The deficiency of which hormone(s) results in mental retardation:
   a growth hormone. b thyroid hormones. c androgens. d estrogen.
4 An increase in the secretion of hypothalamic somatostatin results in
   a the stimulation of protein anabolism.
   b the stimulation of growth.
   c the increased secretion of somatomedins from the liver.
   d the increased secretion of growth hormone.
5 The single criterion for defining true growth is
   a increase in size.
   b increase in weight.
   c formation and elimination of waste products.
   d increased synthesis and accumulation of protein.
   e increased utilization of growth hormone.

Module IV • Energy expenditure and caloric balance

OBJECTIVES

Upon completion of this module, the student will be able to:

1 State the first law of thermodynamics and apply the equation E = heat + work to the concept of metabolic rate.
2 Define and distinguish between *internal* and *external work.*
3 Describe energy balance by stating the formula: total energy expenditure = heat produced + external work + energy storage.
4 Define *metabolic rate;* describe how it is measured directly and indirectly.
5 Define *basal metabolic rate* (*BMR*); distinguish between the terms metabolic rate and basal metabolic rate.
6 Identify the appropriate units of measurement for BMR.
7 Describe *metabolic cost of living.*
8 Define *specific dynamic action* (*SDA*).
9 List and describe the factors that influence metabolic rate (see Table 15-1, p. 536).
10 State the overall energy balance formula as food energy intake = internal heat produced + external work + energy storage.
11 Describe what happens when food intake is greater than or less than the total energy expenditure.
12 Describe the evidence in favor of body energy content being regulated.
13 List the signals that provide short-term and long-term information about the body's energy stores.
14 Define *satiety signals.*
15 Define *obesity* and name its ultimate cause.
16 List the factors that contribute to obesity.
17 Describe the interaction between diet and exercise in the maintenance of body weight.
18 Describe how early-life overfeeding may predispose an individual to adult obesity.
19 Describe the syndrome *anorexia nervosa.*

READING ASSIGNMENT

Chap. 15, pp. 533–542.

EXERCISES

Directions: Answer the following questions in the space provided.

1 You are going to determine the basal metabolic rate (BMR) of a patient. Name
535 three conditions that are necessary to determine the BMR.

a ____________________

____

b ____________________

____

c ____________________

____

2 Would the metabolic rate of the same subject, when not in the postabsorptive state, be higher or lower than above? Why? **536**

____

____

____

3 Write an equation for the total energy expenditure of the body. Under what conditions does food intake equal the internal heat production and external work? **537–538**

____

____

____

4 Describe how to determine the metabolic rate of an individual by indirect calorimetry. **534–535**

____

____

____

5 Listed below are 10 factors that affect food intake. For each, state whether the factor inhibits (I) or stimulates (S) eating. **540**

a increased plasma glucose ______

b increased plasma insulin ______

c increased plasma glucagon ______

d increased cholecystokinin ______

e increased body temperature ______

f increased plasma glycerol ______

g activation of stretch and chemoreceptors in stomach and duodenum ______

h conditioned responses ______

i stress ______

j increased palatability of food ______

SELF-TEST

Directions: Circle the correct answer(s).

1 Which of these factors can significantly change the metabolic rate?

a emotions
b clothing
c muscle tone
d exercise

e SDA
f aging
g surface area of body
h pregnancy

2 A woman is approximately 50 lb overweight. What else can be said for sure about this individual?
   a She has a lower metabolic rate than normal.
   b She eats more than the average person.
   c She has an emotional problem.
   d She has a poor heat-control mechanism.
   e She is suffering from hyperthyroidism.
   f If she continued her present eating habits, she could still lose weight.
   g In the equation for overall energy balance, she has an energy storage term that is negative.
3 Which of the following signals would lead to increased food intake?
   a increased plasma glucose concentration
   b increased plasma insulin concentration
   c increased plasma glucagon concentration
   d a rise in body temperature
   e a rise in cholecystokinin concentration
4 In determining the *metabolic rate* of an individual by *indirect calorimetry*
   a the heat lost from the individual is determined.
   b the amount of oxygen consumed per unit time is measured.
   c an estimate of 1 kcal/4.8 L of oxygen is used.
   d the person *must* be at rest in a room at comfortable temperature and have not eaten for at least 12 h.

Module V • Regulation of body temperature

OBJECTIVES

Upon completion of this module, the student will be able to:

1 Identify the adaptive significance of *homeothermy.*
2 Describe the normal range and variations in body temperature.
3 Identify the physiological sources of heat production.
4 Describe the mechanisms of heat loss, including a discussion of *radiation, conduction, convection,* and *evaporation,* and their relation to blood flow and to behavioral changes.
5 State how evaporation from the body surface and from the linings of the respiratory tract results in heat loss; describe the relationship between relative humidity and evaporation.

6 Describe the effector mechanisms that decrease or increase heat loss and those that decrease or increase heat production.
7 Describe the neural pathways that coordinate temperature regulation, including *thermoreceptors* (central and peripheral) and the brain areas that integrate this information.
8 Identify the exocrine and endocrine mechanisms allowing *acclimatization* to high temperatures.
9 Define *fever.*
10 Describe the role of *endogenous pyrogen* and *prostaglandins* in resetting the brain's "thermostat."
11 Contrast *hyperthermia* with fever.
12 Describe the effect of exercise on body temperature and on the "set point" temperature.
13 Describe the conditions *heat exhaustion* and *heat stroke.*

READING ASSIGNMENT

Chap. 12, pp. 542–550.

EXERCISES

PART I

Directions: Answer the following questions in the space provided.

1 What is the adaptive significance of homeothermy? **542**

____

____

____

2 Describe the thermoregulatory effects of warming or cooling the hypothalamus or skin. **547–548**

____

____

____

3 Describe the effects of continued exposure to a warm environment on the onset of sweating and the composition of the sweat. **548**

____

____

____

4 Describe the fundamental difference between the elevation in body temperature observed during fever with the elevation in body temperature that accompanies
549–550 exercise.

____

____

____

5 Contrast the activity of the thermoregulatory systems in heat exhaustion and heat
550 stroke.

____

____

____

PART II

Directions: Supply the information needed to complete the following chart. Try to sup-
547 ply at least one example for each of the spaces.

	Voluntary Behavior	Physiological Change
In response to cold:		
To decrease heat loss		
To increase heat production		
In response to heat:		
To increase heat loss		
To decrease heat production		

SELF-TEST

PART I

Directions: Circle the correct answer(s).

1 On entering a cold environment
  a our peripheral blood vessels become vasoconstricted.
  b we increase our production of sweat.
  c our muscle tone decreases.
  d our basal metabolic rate increases.
  e we increase our skin surface area.

2 In a hot environment
  a vasoconstriction of our skin blood vessels occurs.
  b after several days, our production of sweat has increased and the sodium content has decreased.
  c we voluntarily decrease our activity.

d our hypothalamus receives information about the high environmental temperature from peripheral receptors in the skin.

3 Which of the following statements are true concerning heat loss by evaporation?
   a Evaporation of water is most efficient in a humid environment.
   b Increased activity of sympathetic nerves increases the sweat rate.
   c At high environmental temperatures, people tend to gain heat from their surroundings by evaporation.
   d Human beings do not evaporate water from their respiratory tract.

4 Heating the hypothalamus of an experimental animal (e.g., the dog) will result in
   a panting.
   b peripheral vasodilation.
   c shivering.
   d fluffing the fur and curling up.

5 A fever
   a results in a person's regulation of body temperature at a higher level.
   b results from an inability to maintain a normal body temperature.
   c is similar to heat stroke in that they are both a result in the breakdown in function of the temperature regulatory centers.
   d results from the internal production of a substance known as endogenous pyrogen.

6 During heat stroke
   a body temperature is regulated at a higher "thermostat setting."
   b in the face of a rapidly rising body temperature, sweat rate declines.
   c as body temperature rises, heat production also rises.
   d as a result of *negative*-feedback control, body temperature returns to normal.

PART II

Directions: Circle T for true and F for false.

T F 1 A desert nomad would have a higher salt content in his sweat than an Eskimo.

T F 2 As the external environmental temperature drops, reflex controls increase peripheral vasoconstriction.

T F 3 A prostaglandin might lead to fever by causing a *depression* in the hypothalamic "set-point" or "thermostat setting."

T F 4 Infections lead to the inability of the body to regulate its temperature and thus cause fevers.

T F 5 Aspirin is an inhibitor of prostaglandin synthesis.

Answers

CHAPTER 15 • MODULE I

1 a, b, c, d (511)
2 a, b, c, d (511–512)
3 a, b, c (508)
4 a (508–509)
5 a (510–511)
6 a, b, c, d (505–506)
7 c (510–512)

CHAPTER 15 • MODULE II

PART I

1 aA, bD, cF, dB (513)
2 glucose, amino acid (515)
3 urine (517)
4 insulin (518)
5 a decreases (513)
 b increases (519)
 c increases (521)
 d increases (523)
 e increases (523)
6 hypoglycemia (524)
7 low-density lipoproteins or LDL (526)
8 saturated, bile acids (528)

PART II

1 b, c, d (513–514)
2 a, b, c (516–517)
3 b, c, d (516)
4 a, b, c, d (519–520)
5 a, b (521)
6 None is correct (523)
7 b, c (525)
8 None is correct (528)

CHAPTER 15 • MODULE III

1 c (533)
2 a (530)
3 b (531)
4 None is correct (530–532)
5 d (529)

CHAPTER 15 • MODULE IV

1 a, b, c, d, e, f, g, h (536)
2 f (540–541)
3 c (540)
4 b (Note: d is incorrect because these conditions are for determining an individuals' *basal* metabolic rate) (534–535)

CHAPTER 15 • MODULE V

PART I

1 a (d is incorrect because our metabolic rate increases, not our *basal* metabolic rate) (547)
2 b, c, d (546–549)
3 b (546–547)
4 a, b (547–548)
5 a, d (549)
6 b, c (550)

PART II

1 F (Part of acclimation to heat is a lower sodium content in sweat, which results in a reduced salt loss.) (549)
2 T (547)
3 F (The fever is caused by an elevation of the temperature "set point.") (549)
4 F (549)
5 T (549)

16
REPRODUCTION

Module I • Male reproductive physiology
Module II • Female reproductive physiology
Module III • Pregnancy
Module IV • Sex development

Module I • Male reproductive physiology

OBJECTIVES

Upon completion of this module, the student will be able to:

1 Define *gonad*, *ovary*, *testis*, *gametes*, *germ cells*, *meiosis*, *zygote*, *accessory reproductive organ*, *secondary sexual characteristics*.
2 Differentiate between *puberty* and *adolescence*.
3 Describe the two major functions of the testes.
4 Describe the role of *gonadotropin-releasing hormone* (*GnRH*) and the *pituitary gonadotropins* (*FSH and LH*) in gametogenesis and sex hormone secretion.
5 Describe the anatomical organization of the male reproductive tract including the terms *scrotum*, *testis*, *seminiferous tubules*, *interstitial cells*, *epididymis*, *vas deferens*, *ejaculatory duct*, *urethra*, *bulbourethral gland*, *seminal vesicles*, and *prostate gland*.
6 Describe *spermatogenesis*, including the terms *spermatogonia*, *primary spermatocyte*, *secondary spermatocyte*, *spermatid*, and *spermatozoa*.
7 Contrast *mitosis* and *meiosis* in terms of location and numbers of chromosomes present after the final division.
8 Describe the role of *crossing over* in passage of genetic material to potential offspring.
9 Describe the role of the *acrosome* in fertilization.
10 Describe the location and list the functions of the *Sertoli cells*.

11 Describe the route that sperm must travel from the seminiferous tubules to outside the body.
12 Describe the *maturation process* of sperm and identify its location.
13 List the constituents of *semen*.
14 Describe the vascular mechanism for producing *erection* in the male; describe the neural control of the erectile tissue of the penis.
15 Define *impotence*.
16 Describe *ejaculation*; list the receptors and afferent and efferent pathways involved.
17 Define *emission* and *orgasm*.
18 Name the anterior pituitary gonadotropins that control testicular function; state their effects on spermatogenesis and testosterone secretion.
19 Describe the negative-feedback control of pituitary gonadotropins caused by secretion of *inhibin* and *testosterone*.
20 List the effects of testosterone and other *androgens*.
21 Define *vasectomy*; describe how this results in sterilization.
22 Define *secondary sex characteristics*.
23 Describe the relationship of *dihydrotestosterone* and *estrogen* (*estradiol*) to testosterone.
24 Describe the permissive effects of *prolactin*.

READING ASSIGNMENT

Chap. 16, pp. 551–565.

EXERCISES

PART I

554 Directions: On Fig. W-23, label the following items:

1 testes
2 seminal vesicle
3 epididymis
4 vas deferens
5 urethra
6 bulbourethral gland
7 prostate gland
8 ejaculatory duct

PART II

Directions: Define the following terms.

1 zygote ____________________

552 ____________________

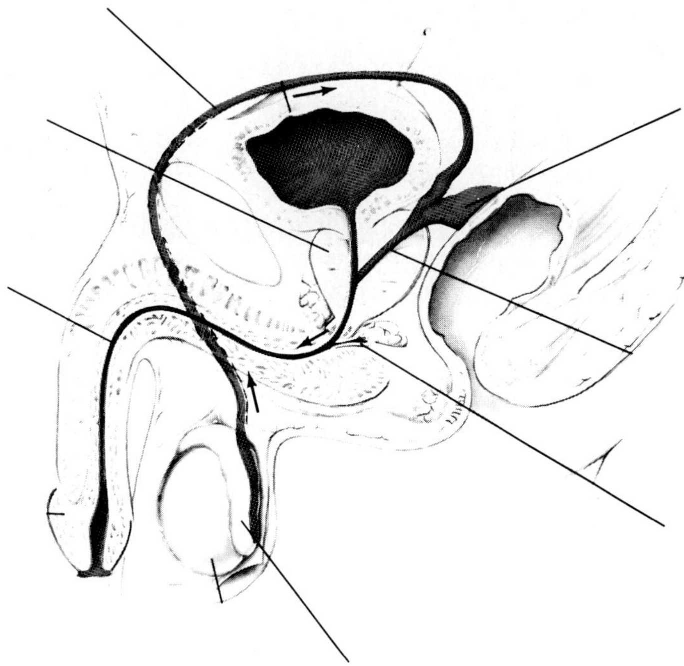

Fig. W-23

2 puberty ______________________________

______________________________ **552**

3 adolescence ______________________________

______________________________ **552**

4 acrosome ______________________________

______________________________ **554**

5 semen ______________________________

______________________________ **558**

6 impotence ______________________________

______________________________ **560**

7 emission ______________________________

______________________________ **560**

8 androgens ______________________________

______________________________ **563**

9 vasectomy ______________________________

______________________________ **564**

10 accessory reproductive organs ______

564 ______

PART III

Directions: Answer the following questions in the space provided.

558–560 1 Describe the vascular mechanisms and neural control of erection.

______

______

______

559 2 List five functions of the Sertoli cells.

a ______

______

b ______

______

c ______

______

d ______

______

e ______

______

562 3 What is the effect of low FSH secretion on spermatogenesis?

______

______

______

4 Describe how a vasectomy can result in sterilization without affecting secondary
564 sexual characteristics.

______

______

______

563–564 5 List the effects of testosterone and other androgens.

______

____

____

SELF-TEST

PART I

Directions: Complete the following items in the space provided.

1 The production of sperm is called ______________________.

2 Ejaculation is usually accompanied by intense pleasure known as ______________.

3 Undifferentiated germ cells from males are called ______________________.

4 During meiosis, genetic material can exchange between maternal and paternal chromosomes by a process known as ______________________.

5 Spermatids have ________ (number) nonduplicated chromosomes.

6 The bulk of the fluid secretions in semen come from the ______________________, ______________________, and ______________________ glands.

7 The cells that secrete testosterone are the ______________________.

8 The hypothalamic-releasing factor for FSH and LH is called ______________.

9 The hormone ______________________, which comes from the testes, inhibits FSH secretion.

10 Three pituitary hormones are known to affect reproductive function in males. They are FSH, LH, and ______________________.

PART II

Directions: Circle the correct answer(s).

1 During spermatogenesis
  a four primary spermatocytes are formed from each spermatogonium.
  b four secondary spermatocytes are formed from each spermatogonium.
  c each mature spermatozoa has 23 chromosomes.
  d each spermatogonium has 23 chromosomes.

2 Which of the following are true of erection in the male?
  a During excitation, the arterioles in the penis constrict.
  b During erection, the veins emptying from the penis constrict.
  c Sympathetic nerves to the arterioles of the penis are stimulated.
  d Parasympathetic nerves to the arterioles of the penis are stimulated.

3 Which of the following are true of ejaculation in the male?
  a It has an afferent pathway similar to that for erection.

b Sperm are able to leak into the bladder.
c It results from contraction of smooth muscle only.
d It is followed by a latent period during which erection is impossible.

4 In the human male
a sperm are stored in the epididymis and in the first part of the vas deferens before ejaculation.
b spermatogenesis occurs in the seminiferous tubules.
c a vasectomy is performed to terminate spermatogenesis.
d following castration the accessory reproductive organs decrease in size.

5 The Sertoli cells
a nourish developing sperm.
b produce testosterone.
c secrete the hormone inhibin.
d secrete fluid into the lumen of the seminiferous tubules.

6 Possible causes of deficient erection and ejaculation, decreased size in reproductive organs, and inhibition of smooth muscle activities in the ducts in the adult male could be
a increased LH secretion.
b high testosterone secretion.
c removal of the anterior pituitary.
d castration.

7 In some target cells testosterone undergoes a transformation to
a progesterone.
b luteinizing hormone.
c estrogen.
d dihydrotestosterone.

8 A lesion in the hypothalamus that destroyed the area responsible for secretion of GnRH would cause
a inhibition of testosterone secretion.
b excessive beard growth.
c increased production of sperm.
d cyclical release of LH secretion.

Module II • Female reproductive physiology

OBJECTIVES

Upon completion of this module, the student will be able to:

1 Label the following items on a diagram of the ovaries and other female reproductive structures: ovary, fimbriae, uterine tube (oviduct), uterus, cervix, vagina, clitoris, hymen, labia majora, labia minora.

2 Describe the structure and function of the following ovarian structures: *primary follicle, maturing follicle, zona pellucida, ovum, granulosa cells, theca, antrum, cumulus oophorus.*
3 Define *ovulation.*
4 Describe the mitotic and meiotic divisions of the ovum; contrast ovum development (*oogenesis*) with spermatogenesis.
5 Describe the formation of the corpus luteum.
6 Name the ovarian hormones; state their chemical nature and site of origin.
7 Mark the *follicular phase*, the *luteal phase*, and the day of ovulation on a scale of 28 days, beginning with day 1 as the first day of menstrual bleeding.
8 State the changes in LH, FSH, estrogen, and progesterone throughout the 28-day menstrual cycle; describe what causes these changes.
9 Diagram the *negative-* and *positive-feedback* effects of inhibin, estrogen, and progesterone on GnRH, FSH,and LH secretion.
10 Describe the hormonal control of ovulation.
11 State the factors responsible for the LH peak in midcycle.
12 Describe the function and control of the corpus luteum.
13 Define *myometrium* and *endometrium.*
14 Identify the *menstrual, proliferative,* and *secretory phases* on a 28-day scale, beginning with day 1 as the first day of menstrual bleeding.
15 Describe the changes in uterine endometrium during the menstrual cycle; explain them in terms of the hormonal patterns.
16 State the major cause of *dysmenorrhea.*
17 State the nonuterine effects of estrogen and progesterone.
18 Describe the female sexual response.
19 State the hormone controlling sex drive in the female.

READING ASSIGNMENT

Chap. 16, pp. 566–580.

EXERCISES

PART I

Directions: Fig. W-24 shows the secretion patterns of a woman's hormones. Label the following items. 572

1 LH pattern of fluctuation
2 FSH pattern of fluctuation
3 secretion paterns of estrogen
4 secretion patterns of progesterone
5 follicular phase of cycle
6 menstrual flow
7 the point of ovulation
8 luteal phase of cycle
9 proliferative phase of cycle
10 secretory phase of cycle

PART II

Directions: Answer the following questions in the space provided.

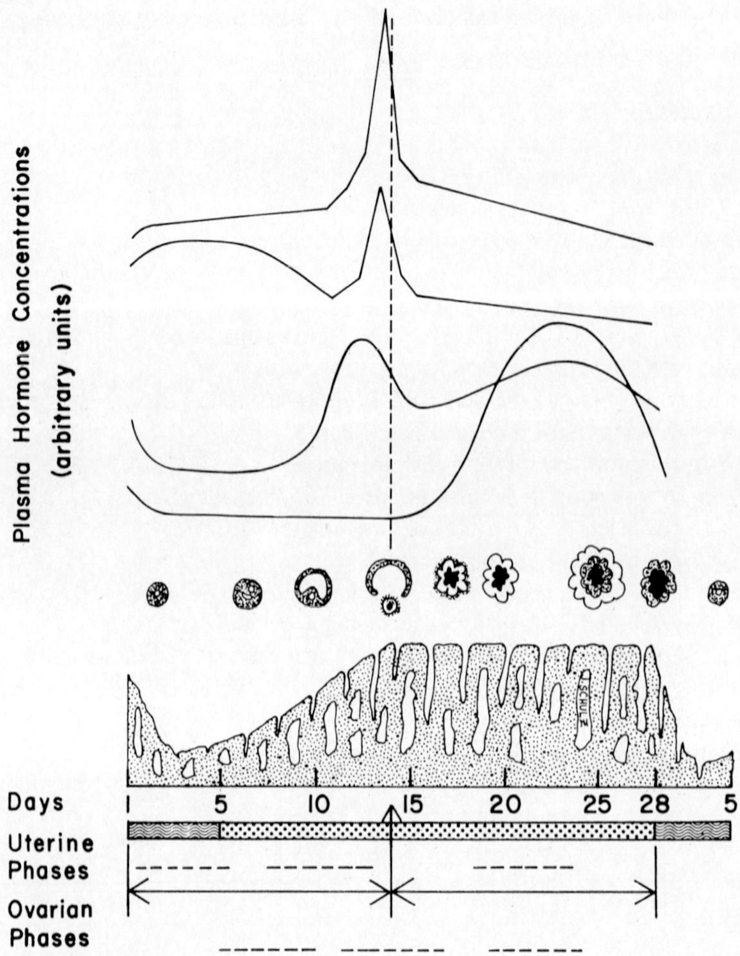

Fig. W-24

1 Indicate with an ↑ for increase and ↓ for decrease the effects of the following com-
binations of ovarian hormones on the secretion of GnRH and on the pituitary's
574 secretion of FSH and LH.

a low plasma estrogen

GnRH secretion ____________________

FSH secretion ____________________

LH secretion ____________________

b high plasma estrogen

GnRH secretion ____________________

LH secretion ____________________

FSH secretion ____________________

c high plasma progesterone in presence of estrogen — GnRH secretion ____________

LH secretion ____________

FSH secretion ____________

d secretion of inhibin — LH secretion ____________

FSH secretion ____________

2 Describe the stages of ovum development. **567–570**

____

____

____

____

3 State the multiple effects of prostaglandins on the female reproductive system. **576**

____

____

____

____

____

SELF-TEST

PART I

Directions: Circle the correct answer(s).

1 Ovulation results from a midcycle increase in
 a FSH. b LH. c estrogen. d progesterone.

2 Progesterone secretion is highest during which of the following phases?
 a follicular b luteal c proliferative d menstrual flow

3 Follicle and ovum development is dependent on the presence of
 a FSH. b LH. c estrogen. d progesterone.

4 A decrease in blood estrogen and progesterone levels, resulting from degeneration of the corpus luteum, leads to what endometrial changes?
 a release of vasoconstrictor prostaglandins that decrease uterine blood flow
 b the proliferative phase
 c menstruation
 d the secretory phase

5 The corpus luteum
 a forms from the ruptured follicle.
 b degenerates within 24 h of ovulation unless the ovum is fertilized.

c secretes both estrogen and progesterone.
d is present during the follicular phase of the menstrual cycle.

6 High plasma levels of estrogen that are present during the late follicular phase
a stimulate the hypothalamus to secrete GnRH.
b act on the pituitary gland and result in increased sensitivity to GnRH.
c have a positive-feedback effect on LH secretion.
d have a negative-feedback effect on LH secretion.

7 The LH surge
a occurs during the secretory phase of the menstrual cycle.
b is in response to high plasma levels of progesterone.
c occurs about day 28 of the menstrual cycle.
d occurs shortly after ovulation.

8 High plasma estrogen
a stimulates the growth of uterine smooth muscle (myometrium).
b inhibits the growth of uterine glandular epithelium (endometrium).
c causes fluid retention.
d leads to growth of ovaries and follicles.

9 High plasma progesterone
a in conjunction with estrogen has a positive-feedback effect on GnRH.
b in conjunction with estrogen leads to an increased secretion of FSH and LH.
c stimulates the growth of the myometrium during pregnancy.
d results in an increased frequency of ovulation.

10 Which of the following statements are true concerning the female sexual response?
a It is characterized by marked vasocongestion.
b Orgasm is essential to fertilization.
c Libido is reduced following removal of the ovaries.
d Libido is reduced following removal of the adrenal glands.

PART II

Directions: Circle T for true and F for false.

T F 1 Sex drive in the female is thought to be controlled mainly by blood levels of estrogen.

T F 2 Myometrium is the smooth muscle layer of the uterus.

T F 3 Progesterone is secreted in increasingly large amounts as the follicle develops.

T F 4 One nonuterine effect of estrogen is the development of secondary sexual characteristics.

T F 5 It is the increase in progesterone near the end of the cycle that leads to menstruation.

T F 6 The antrum is the fluid-filled space found in the developing follicle.

T F 7 In contrast to spermatogenesis, during oogenesis (ovum development), each primitive ovum produces only one mature ovum containing 23 chromosomes.

PART III

Directions: Using Fig. W-25, a composite diagram of hormonal and other events in the menstrual cycle, label the

1 LH pattern of secretion.
2 FSH pattern of secretion.
3 secretion pattern of estrogen.
4 secretion pattern of progesterone.
5 proliferative phase.
6 secretory phase.
7 follicular phase
8 luteal phase.
9 point of ovulation.

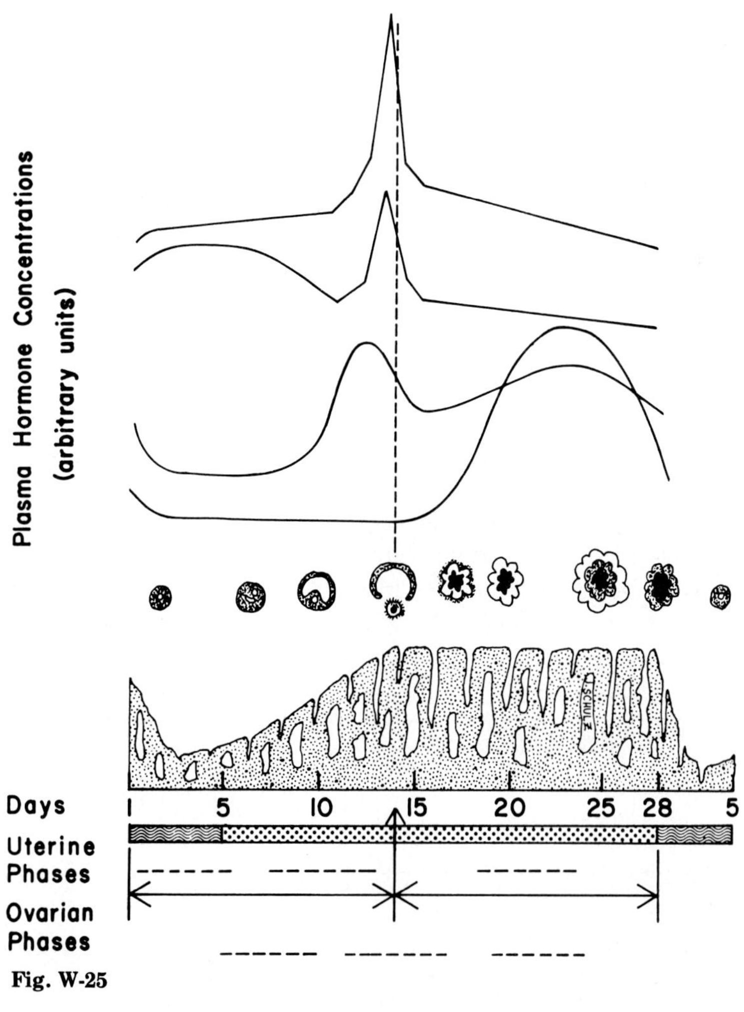

Fig. W-25

Module III • Pregnancy

OBJECTIVES

Upon completion of this module, the student will be able to:

1 State the duration of sperm and ovum viability after ejaculation and ovulation.
2 Describe transport of the ovum from ovary to uterus.
3 Describe transport of sperm from vagina to oviduct.
4 Describe sperm *capacitation* and *activation*.
5 Describe the entry of the sperm into the ovum.
6 Describe the early development of the fertilized ovum and its implantation, and the process of placentation, including descriptions of the *blastocyst*, *embryoblast*, *trophoblast*, *placenta*, *embryo*, and *fetus*.
7 Describe the function of the *umbilical arteries* and *veins* and the *amniotic cavity*.
8 Describe the hormonal changes during pregnancy.
9 Describe the chemical nature of *chorionic gonadotropin* (*CG*), its site of synthesis, stimuli for release, effector organs, and effect.
10 Describe the basis of the CG pregnancy test.
11 Describe the site of synthesis and the physiological effects of *estriol* and *placental lactogen*.
12 Define *toxemia of pregnancy*.
13 Describe *labor*, *parturition*, *afterbirth*, and the accompanying hormonal changes.
14 Describe how intrauterine position of the baby can complicate parturition.
15 Predict the effects on uterine motility of secretion of progesterone, release of oxytocin, and injection of prostaglandins.
16 Describe the glandular structure of the breasts and the hormonal influences that act on them.
17 Describe the control of prolactin secretion during nursing.
18 Describe the *milk let-down reflex*; identify the stimuli, receptors, afferent and efferent pathways, integrating center, effector organ, and reflex response.
19 Describe the primary means of preventing pregnancy and their relative effectiveness.

READING ASSIGNMENT

Chap. 16, pp. 580–591.

EXERCISES

PART I

Directions: Answer the following questions in the space provided.

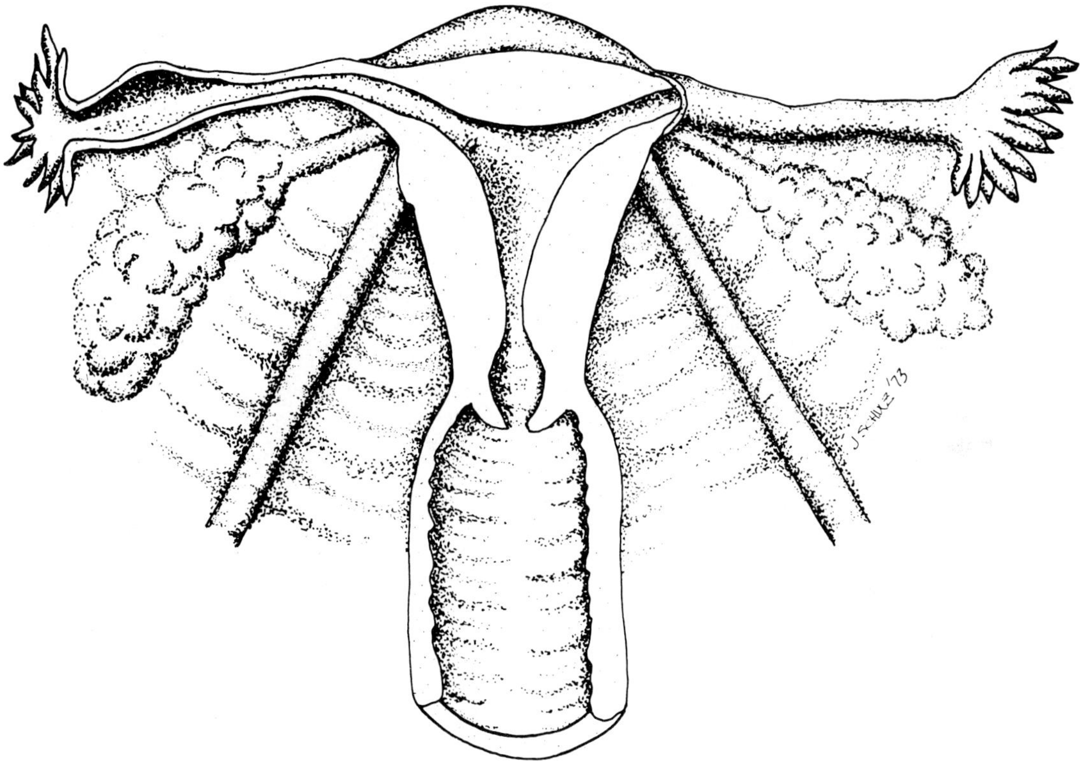

Fig. W-26: Female reproductive system.

1 On a diagram of the female internal reproductive organs (Fig. W-26) show (using arrows) the routes of sperm and ovum movement, the average times for movement, the normal site of fertilization, and the normal site for implantation of the blastocyst (developing embryo). **567, 580–581**

2 List the effects of the following hormones on parturition. **588–589**

a progesterone ______________________________

____

b oxytocin ______________________________

____

c prostaglandins ______________________________

____

3 List the effects of the following hormones on mammary-gland development and lactation. **589–590**

a estrogen ______________________________

____

b progesterone ______________________________

____

c prolactin-inhibiting hormone ______________________________

____

d prolactin ______________________________

____

e placental lactogen ______________________________

____

f oxytocin ______________________________

____

589–590 4 Describe the neural control of prolactin secretion during suckling.

____

____

____

____

591 5 Describe the scientific basis of oral contraceptives.

____

____

____

SELF-TEST

Directions: Circle the correct answer(s).

1 Which of the following are correct concerning early development, implantation, and placentation?
  a It takes approximately 2 to 3 weeks for the fertilized ovum to move through the oviduct to the uterus.
  b Implantation of the fertilized ovum takes place on about day 7 of the menstrual cycle.
  c The embryo is called a fetus after the end of the 5th or 6th month of development.
  d At the time of implantation, the fertilized ovum has developed into a ball of cells called a blastocyst.

2 For fertilization to occur
  a the sperm must have its surface layer of glycoproteins removed, a process known as activation.
  b the activated sperm loses its tail while still in the epididymis.
  c the nuclei of the sperm and ovum must unite.
  d the sperm's plasma membrane must fuse with the ovum's plasma membrane.

3 During pregnancy
  a steroid hormones such as estrogen and progesterone are produced by the corpus luteum during the first 2 months.
  b the placenta produces a hormone called chorionic gonadotropin.
  c chorionic gonadotropin stimulates steroid secretion by the corpus luteum.
  d removal of the corpus luteum at any time results in abortion.

4 Parturition
  a is induced by an increase in secretion of progesterone.
  b can be induced by an injection of oxytocin.
  c can be induced by an injection of prostaglandin.

5 Which of the following statements are true concerning lactation and breast development?
  a Estrogen stimulates duct growth and breast enlargement.
  b Prolactin secretion during pregnancy can lead to enlargement of the breasts.
  c Prolactin inhibits milk production.
  d Oxytocin results in milk "let-down."

6 Which of the following statements are true concerning birth control?
  a Oral contraceptives generally block the LH surge.
  b Oral contraceptives always prevent ovulation.
  c The intrauterine device blocks the LH surge.
  d The intrauterine device may work by preventing implantation of the blastocyst.

Module IV • Sex development

OBJECTIVES

Upon completion of this module, the student will be able to:

1 State the genetic difference between males and females.
2 Define *sex differentiation.*
3 Describe the differentiation of the gonads, including a discussion of the *H-Y antigen.*
4 Describe the differentiation of internal and external genitalia.
5 State the effects of testosterone and *Müllerian inhibitory substance* (*MIS*) on differentiation of the genitalia.

6 State the inherent problem in the syndrome *testicular feminization.*
7 Explain what is meant by sexual differentiation of the central nervous system.
8 Define *puberty*; describe the hormonal events involved in it.
9 Define *precocious puberty.*
10 Define *menarche.*
11 Describe the physical and hormonal changes during *menopause* and *climacteric.*
12 Describe the sexual changes in males in aging.

READING ASSIGNMENT

Chap. 16, pp. 592–598.

EXERCISES

PART I

Directions: Match the words in Column A with the characteristics in Column B by placing the appropriate letter in the space provided.

Column A			Column B
1 ______	Müllerian duct	**593**	a protein secreted by males
2 ______	Wolffian ducts	**593**	b persists in females
			c persists in males
3 ______	testicular feminization	**593**	d caused by lack of androgen receptors
4 ______	H-Y antigen	**593**	e first menstrual period
			f last menstrual period
5 ______	menopause	**597**	g cessation of reproductive function
6 ______	menarche	**597**	
7 ______	climacteric	**598**	

PART II

Directions: Answer the following questions in the space provided.

1 Describe the differences between estrogen secretion and gonadotropin secretion
597 in a woman 25 years of age and one who has gone through menopause.

____

____

____

2 Describe what is meant by the expression "The early fetus is sexually bipoten-
593 tial."

____

3 Describe evidence that there are distinct "male" and "female" brains. **595**

4 Describe the role of the X and Y chromosomes in determining the sex of an individual. **592**

SELF-TEST

Directions: Circle the correct answer(s).

1 Which of the following statements are correct concerning the differentiation of the internal and external genitalia?
   a If the area from which the gonads will derive is removed in the early fetus, then the gonadless embryo will develop the female duct system.
   b Normally, the presence of testes represses the development of the female duct system.
   c When testosterone is present, the embryological development follows the female pattern.
   d It is possible to have internal and external genitalia of different sexes if there is a failure in the gonadal hormone secretion at a critical period.

2 Which of the following statements are true concerning sexual differentiation of the central nervous system?
   a Genetic female monkeys given testosterone during late fetal life have masculinized external genitalia.
   b Genetic female monkeys given testosterone during late fetal life have masculine sex behavior as adults.
   c Genetic female monkeys given testosterone during late fetal life have masculine play-type behavior during growth.
   d Studies on people indicate that the most important factor determining gender identity is in utero exposure to male or female hormones.

3 Puberty
   a in males is a result of the onset of increased testosterone secretion by the testes.
   b in males is associated with increased GnRH secretion.
   c in females is a direct result of an increased secretion of progesterone by the ovaries.
   d in females is associated with increased GnRH secretion.

4 Menopause
  a results in increased secretion of estrogen.
  b results in an increased likelihood of developing atherosclerosis.
  c results in an increased frequency of menstrual periods.
  d results in an increased secretion of gonadotropins.

Answers

CHAPTER 16 • MODULE I

PART I

1 spermatogenesis (553)
2 orgasm (560)
3 spermatogonia (553)
4 crossing over (554)
5 23 (557)
6 prostate, seminal vesicles, bulbourethral (558)
7 interstitial cells (553)
8 gonadotropin-releasing hormone (GnRH) (552)
9 inhibin (563)
10 prolactin (565)

PART II

1 b, c (557)
2 b, d (559–560)
3 a, d (560–561)
4 a, b, d (553, 564)
5 a, c, d (559)
6 c, d (561–564)
7 c, d (565)
8 a (562–564)

CHAPTER 16 • MODULE II

PART I

1 b (574)
2 b (572)
3 a, b, c (572–573)
4 a, c (577)
5 a, c (570, 575–576)
6 a, b, c (574)
7 None is correct (574)
8 a, c, d (576–578)
9 c (574, 578)
10 a, d (579)

PART II

1 F (579)
2 T (576)
3 F (572)
4 T (578)
5 F (577)
6 T (568)
7 T (570)

PART III

See Fig. 16-18, p. 572

CHAPTER 16 • MODULE III

1 d (581–582)
2 c, d (580–581)
3 b, c, d (584–585)
4 b, c (588)
5 a, b, d (589–590)
6 a, d (591)

CHAPTER 16 • MODULE IV

1 a, b, d (593)
2 a, b, c (594–595)
3 a, b, d (595–596)
4 b, d (597–598)

17

DEFENSE MECHANISMS OF THE BODY: IMMUNOLOGY, FOREIGN CHEMICALS, AND STRESS

Module I • Immunology: effector cells and nonspecific immune responses

OBJECTIVES

Upon completion of this module, the student will be able to:

1 Define *immunity* and *immune surveillance.*
2 Distinguish between *specific* and *nonspecific immune responses.*
3 List the major types of foreign material encountered by the immune system.
4 List the major effector-cell types of the immune system, their primary sites of production, and their primary functions.
5 Define and list the location of *lymphoid tissues.*
6 State the functions of the *lymph nodes, spleen,* and the *thymus.*
7 List the external anatomic and chemical defenses against infection.

8 List the sequence of events in an *inflammatory response.*
9 State the role of *histamine* and the *kinins* in inflammation.
10 Describe the adaptive value of vasodilation and increased permeability that occur during inflammation.
11 Describe the *chemotactic* response of neutrophils to inflammation.
12 Describe the process of *phagocytosis,* including a description of *degranulation* and the *phagolysosome.*
13 Describe the role of *lactoferrin, natural killer cells,* and the *complement system* in direct killing of microbes.
14 Differentiate between an *abscess* and a *granuloma.*
15 Describe the *complement cascade system.*
16 Describe the role of the *membrane attack complex* (*MAC*) in the killing of foreign cells.
17 List the multiple effects of activation of *complement proteins.*
18 Contrast the *classic complement pathway* with the *alternate pathway.*
19 Describe the role of *endogenous pyrogen* (*EP*), *leukocyte endogenous mediator* (*LEM*), and *interleukin 1* (*IL-1*) in the systemic manifestation of inflammation.
20 Define and describe the effects of *interferon.*

READING ASSIGNMENT

Chap. 17, pp. 599–613.

EXERCISES

Directions: Answer the following questions in the space provided.

600 1 What is the difference between specific and nonspecific immune responses?

2 After each of the following effector cells of the immune system, list its primary
601 site of production and primary known function.

a macrophages

b monocytes

c plasma cells

d lymphocytes ______

______

e neutrophils ______

______

f basophils ______

______

g eosinophils ______

______

3 List the sequence of events in an inflammatory response, beginning with

a initial entry of bacteria or other foreign substance, and ending with (g) tissue repair. 604

b ______

c ______

d ______

e ______

f ______

4 Describe the adaptive value of the vascular changes that occur with inflammation. 604

______

______

______

5 Describe the structures and chemicals involved in the killing of phagocytized microorganisms. 606–607

______

______

______

6 Neutrophils and macrophages function in the inflammatory process not only as phagocytes but also as secretory cells. List the multiple effects of secretions of chemicals by phagocytes on nonspecific immunity. 607–612

______

______

______

609 7 List the effects of the activation of complement proteins.

____

____

____

8 List the effects of the release of EP, LEM, and IL-1 on the systemic manifestations
610–611 of the inflammation.

____

____

____

SELF-TEST

PART I

Directions: Complete the following items in the space provided.

1 Immune responses can be classified into two categories: ________________ and ____________________.

2 Neutrophils, eosinophils, basophils, many lymphocytes, and monocytes are produced in the ____________________.

3 Number (1 through 7) the following sequence of events in a local infection.

a ______ exit of neutrophils (and later monocytes) from the vessels into the tissues

b ______ repair of tissue

c ______ initial entry of microbes

d ______ phagocytosis and destruction of the microbes

e ______ filtration of fluid into the tissues, with resultant swelling

f ______ vasodilation of all vessels of the microcirculation, leading to increased blood flow

g ______ a marked increase in vascular permeability to protein

4 The exposure of the microbe to the digestive enzymes in the lysosome by fusion of the phagosome and lysosome membranes results in a process called ________________________.

5 A(n) ____________________ is a bag of pus containing microbes, leukocytes, and liquified debris walled off by fibroblasts and collagen.

PART II

Directions: Circle the correct answer(s).

1 Which of the following are functions of the spleen?
  a It produces red blood cells in adults.
  b It produces new lymphocytes.
  c It removes products of red blood cell degradation and other foreign matter by macrophage phagocytosis.
  d It stores red blood cells, which can then be added to the circulation.

2 Lymph nodes
  a store red blood cells.
  b add new lymphocytes to lymph flow through the lymph nodes.
  c have macrophages that phagocytize particulate matter.
  d produce antibodies and sensitized T cells.

3 Monocytes
  a are primarily produced in lymph nodes.
  b can secrete endogenous pyrogen.
  c can be converted to macrophages.
  d can secrete interleukin 1.

4 Neutrophils
  a are a type of lymphocyte.
  b are a type of leukocyte.
  c are produced in the bone marrow.
  d can release chemicals involved in inflammation.

5 Which of the following statements are correct concerning the external anatomic and chemical barriers of the nonspecific immune system?
  a Most microorganisms can penetrate the intact skin.
  b The sweat, sebaceous, and lacrimal glands secrete chemical substances that kill many forms of bacteria.
  c Many bacteria that live on the skin and other linings of the body exposed to the external enivronment suppress the growth of virulent microorganisms.
  d Acid secretion in the stomach kills many species of bacteria.

6 Inflammation
  a is a fairly stereotyped response.
  b occurs in response to an injury.
  c results in a decrease in blood flow to the inflamed area.
  d results in a decrease in the capillary permeability in the inflamed area.

7 Which of the following statements are true concerning phagocytosis?
  a The phagocyte engulfs the microorganism by *endocytosis.*
  b Degranulation results in the fusion of the phagosomal membranes with the lysosomal membranes and results in the formation of a phagolysosome.
  c Opsonins are substances that enhance phagocytosis.
  d The phagolysosome produces a high concentration of hydrogen peroxide and other derivatives of oxygen harmful to microorganisms.

8 Which of the following are the result of activation of complement proteins?
  a chemotaxis
  b direct destruction of microbial cells
  c enhancement of phagocytosis
  d vasodilation and increased permeability to proteins

9 The release of EP/LEM/IL-1 during an infection results in
   a the release of acute phase proteins from the liver.
   b a lowering of body temperature.
   c granulopoiesis.
   d lymphocyte proliferation and differentiation.

10 Interferon
   a is a nonspecific defense mechanism, particularly against viral infection.
   b is a protein that is by itself antiviral.
   c occurs in many different forms, each of which is specific for a specific virus.
   d exerts an anticancer effect because most cancers are caused by viruses.

Module II • Immunology: specific immune responses

OBJECTIVES

Upon completion of this module, the student will be able to:

1 Name the two categories of specific immune responses, and list their sites of origin.
2 Define *antigens* and *hapten.*
3 Describe the functions and interactions of B and T cell systems.
4 List the three types of T cells and their primary functions.
5 Define *lymphokines.*
6 Describe the three general interactions of macrophages with B and T cells.
7 List the sequence of events in *humoral immunity* against bacteria.
8 Define *antibody.*
9 List the five classes of *immunoglobulins* and the general functions of each class.
10 Describe the role of *plasma cells, memory cells, clones, macrophages, helper T cells, B-cell growth factor,* and *suppressor T cells* in antibody production.
11 List the amplification functions of antibodies as (a) activation of complement system, (b) direct enhancement of phagocytosis, (c) activation of K cells, and (d) direct neutralization of bacterial toxins and viruses.
12 Contrast *active immunity* with *passive humoral immunity.*
13 Define *cytotoxic T lymphocyte, major histocompatibility complex* (*MHC*), and *human leukocyte associated antigens* (*HLA antigens* or *histocompatibility antigens*).
14 Describe the role of HLA antigens in *cell-mediated immunity.*
15 Contrast cell-mediated immunity with humoral immunity in terms of function, location of plasma cells and sensitized T cells, and amplifications process.
16 Describe the interaction between macrophages and interleukin 1, and helper T lymphocytes and interleukin 2, in the activation of cytotoxic T lymphocytes.

17 Compare and contrast *natural killer cells (NK cells)* with cytotoxic T cells.
18 Describe the interaction of interferon with NK cells, macrophages, and T cells in enhancing defenses against viruses and tumors.
19 Describe the extracellular and intracellular host responses to infection with viruses.
20 Describe the way most cancer cells are normally destroyed (*immune surveillance*).
21 Define and describe *immune enhancement.*
22 Describe the process of tissue-implant *rejection* and methods aimed at its prevention.
23 List the four blood types and the types of antibodies a person will have for each of these blood types.
24 Describe the *Rh-factor* antigens.
25 Describe the effect of *protein-calorie malnutrition* on resistance to infection.
26 Define *antibiotics* and *disinfectants.*
27 Describe the role of *resistance factors* in the generation of antibiotic resistant bacteria.
28 Define *hypersensitivity;* differentiate between *immediate* and *delayed* hypersensitivity.
29 Describe the interactions of *IgE antibodies, mast cells,* and *eosinophils* in immediate hypersensitivity.
30 Define anaphylactic shock.
31 Define *autoimmune disease* and list five possible causes.

READING ASSIGNMENT

Chap. 17, pp. 613–632.

EXERCISES

PART I

Directions: Answer the following questions in the space provided.

1 List the sequence of events in humoral immunity against bacteria. **615**

____

____

____

____

____

2 Describe four functions of antibodies **617–620**

____

____

____

____

618 3 Outline the role of macrophages in the activation, differentiation, and proliferation of B lymphocytes.

621 4 Describe the role of HLA antigens in cell-mediated immunity.

623 5 Outline the role of macrophages in the activation and proliferation of cytotoxic T lymphocytes.

624–625 6 Describe the multiple roles of interferon in defense against cancer cells and viruses.

626–627 7 Why are many tissue transplants destroyed? What would increase the likelihood for a successful transplant? What are the dangers associated with radiation and drug therapy designed to minimize rejection?

629–630 8 Describe the sequence of events leading to an immediate hypersensitivity reaction.

PART II

Directions: Fill in the blanks in the following table. 627

Blood-type Interactions

Recipient	Donor	Compatible?
A	________	yes
______	O, B	yes
O	AB, A, B	______
AB	________	yes
O	O	______
A	AB	______

SELF-TEST

PART I

Directions: Complete the following lines in the space provided.

1 The five classes of immunoglobulins are ______________________________, ______________________________, ______________________________, ______________________________, and ______________________________.

2 B cells are derived from the ______________________________ prior to their taking up residence in lymph nodes and other nonthymic lymphoid tissues.

3 The molecular components of foreign substances that stimulate a specific immune response are called ______________________________.

4 The three types of T cells are ______________________________, ______________________________, and ______________________________.

5 An acquired reactivity to an antigen, which can result in bodily damage on subsequent exposure to that particular antigen, is called ______________________________.

6 The three types of cells that directly attack cancer cells are macrophages, T cells, and ______________________________ cells.

PART II

Directions: Circle the correct answer(s).

1 Antibodies
a are a specialized type of lipid-carbohydrate complex.

b can only bind with protein antigens.
c belong to five classes of immunoglobulins.
d are secreted by plasma cells.

2 Antibody-antigen complexes result in
a amplification of the inflammatory response.
b activation of complement.
c direct enhancement of phagocytosis.
d direct neutralization of bacterial toxins.

3 Active immunity
a is built up as a result of actual contact with microbes or other antigens.
b occurs within minutes of contact with an antigen for the first time.
c generally gives shorter lasting protection than passive immunity.
d is the basis for many types of vaccinations.

4 Cytotoxic T lymphocytes
a are responsible for cell-mediated immunity.
b can release lymphokines.
c can release interferon.
d attack cells that bear a foreign antigen *plus* one of the T cell's own HLA antigens.

5 Which of the following statements are true concerning activation, proliferation, and mechanism of action of cytotoxic T cells?
a Macrophages secrete interleukin 1, which *inhibits* helper T lymphocytes.
b Helper T lymphocytes secrete interleukin 2, which *facilitates* the proliferation of cytotoxic T lymphocytes.
c A *lymphokine* must be secreted for cytotoxic T cells to become activated.
d Once activated, cytotoxic T cells begin to produce and secrete antibodies.

6 Interferon has numerous antiviral and anticancer functions. Among interferons many effects are
a inhibition of natural killer (NK) cells.
b direct inhibition of viral replication.
c stimulation of macrophages.
d stimulation of cytotoxic T cells.

7 Which of the following are true concerning tissue transplants?
a The humoral immune system is mainly responsible for the recognition and rejection of tissue transplants.
b The recipient reacts to histocompatibility antigens found on the transplanted cells.
c The drug cyclosporin is effective in preventing rejection because it blocks T cell proliferation and leaves the B cell system essentially untouched.
d Radiation therapy aimed at increasing transplant success increases the likelihood of developing infections.

8 A person with type B blood
a can receive blood from type O people.
b has antibodies to type B blood.
c has antibodies to type AB blood.
d has antibodies to type O blood.

9 Immediate hypersensitivity
   a does not occur on first exposure to an antigen.
   b is triggered by an antigen stimulating antibody production from the *IgE* class of antibodies.
   c results in the release of large amounts of *antihistamines*.
   d generally results in anaphylactic shock.

10 Which of the following are possible causes of autoimmune disease?
   a Normal antigens may be altered by environmental factors.
   b Genetic mutations may result in new antigens.
   c Prior contact may have been made with microbes with antigens that are close in structure to certain self-antigens.
   d A cell may be infected with a virus with nucleic acid codes for a new protein (antigen).

Module III • Metabolism of foreign chemicals

OBJECTIVES

Upon completion of this module, the student will be able to:

1 Describe the effect of rate of entry, rate of biotransformation, and rate of excretion on the *effective concentration* of any foreign chemical at its sites of action.
2 List the sites of absorption of foreign chemicals.
3 List the major storage sites for foreign chemicals.
4 List the sites of excretion of foreign chemicals.
5 Describe the beneficial and harmful effects of *biotransformation* of foreign chemicals.
6 Define *microsomal enzyme system* (*MES*) and describe its function.
7 Describe the metabolic pathways and harmful effects of alcohol.
8 Describe the effects of the presence of multiple foreign substances on the biotransformation of these substances, using alcohol and barbiturates as an example.

READING ASSIGNMENT

Chap. 17, pp. 632–636.

EXERCISES

Directions: Answer the following questions in the space provided.

634–635 1 Why may biotransformation of some chemicals be harmful?

____

____

____

635–636 2 Describe the effects of ingestion of alcohol on:

A liver function: _______________

____

____

____

B metabolism of other foreign drugs and chemicals when the use of alcohol is:

a short term _______________

____

____

b chronic _______________

____

____

SELF-TEST

Directions: Circle the correct answer(s).

1 Absorption of foreign chemicals can occur through the
   a skin. c gastrointestinal tract.
   b placenta. d lungs.

2 Major storage sites for foreign chemicals are
   a cell proteins. c glycogen in skeletal muscle.
   b bone tissue. d fat depots.

3 Foreign chemicals can be excreted
   a in the feces.
   b in the urine by glomerular filtration.
   c in the urine by tubular secretion.
   d in the air we exhale.

4 Biotransformation of foreign chemicals
   a occurs mainly in the kidneys.
   b can render a chemical either more or less toxic.
   c involves enzymes known as the *macrophage digestive system.*
   d often leads to more lipid-soluble substances.

5 Alcohol biotransformation
 a occurs in the liver.
 b leads to the production of hydrogen and acetaldehyde.
 c results in increased amounts of triacylglycerol in the liver.
 d results in malnutrition, the primary harmful effect of alcohol overuse.

6 The liver microsomal enzyme system
 a always results in the detoxification of chemicals.
 b is an easily inducible system.
 c is a group of enzymes located mainly on the smooth endoplasmic reticulum of liver cells.
 d often results in the metabolism of normal substances found within the body (e.g., steroids).

Module IV • Resistance to stress

OBJECTIVES

Upon completion of this module, the student will be able to:

1 State the responses common to almost all types of stress.
2 Describe the control of cortisol secretion.
3 List the three general effects of cortisol on organic metabolism and state their adaptive value.
4 Describe the effects of cortisol on vascular reactivity.
5 Describe the effects of psychosocial stress on cortisol secretion, and state the possible adaptive value of this response.
6 List the *pharmacological* effects of cortisol.
7 List the seven major effects of increased sympathetic activity during stress.
8 List the other hormones that are released during stress and state their adaptive value.

READING ASSIGNMENT

Chap. 17. pp. 636–640.

EXERCISES

Directions: Complete the following items in the space provided.

1 Identify the effects cortisol has on the following: **637–638**

 a protein catabolism ____________________

 b liver uptake of amino acid ____________________

 c glucose uptake and oxidation ____________________

d gluconeogenesis ______________________

e vascular reactivity ______________________

2 Predict whether cortisol secretion increases, decreases, or remains the same in
638 each of the following situations.

a awaiting a surgical operation ______________________

b sewing ______________________

c during a job interview ______________________

d during sleep ______________________

e eating breakfast ______________________

f during final exams ______________________

639 3 List the seven major effects of increased sympathetic activity in response to stress.

____

____

____

____

____

____

____

SELF-TEST

PART I

Directions: Complete the following items in the space provided.

1 Two responses common to most types of stress are:

a ______________________

b ______________________

2 When cortisol is present in abnormally high concentration, there may appear new effects known as ______________________.

3 Briefly describe the pathway for increased cortisol secretion.

____

____

____

PART II

Directions: Circle the correct answer(s).

1 The cardiovascular response to stress requires
a increased cortisol secretion.

b decreased cortisol secretion.
c no change in cortisol secretion.

2 Large amounts of cortisol may result in
a an increase in antibody production.
b a decrease in antibody production.
c inhibition of phagocytosis.
d inhibition of vasodilation.

3 Which of the following are functions of the sympathetic nervous system during stress?
a decreased glycogenolysis
b increased cardiac output
c redistribution of blood from gastrointestinal tract, kidneys, etc., to skeletal muscle
d increased blood coagulation
e increased adipose-tissue catabolism
f increased skeletal muscle fatigue

4 Which of the following hormones are generally released in greater amounts during stress?
a vasopressin
b aldosterone
c insulin
d glucagon

Answers

CHAPTER 17 • MODULE I

PART I

1 specific, nonspecific (600)
2 bone arrow (601)
3 a 5
b 7
c 1
d 6
e 4
f 2
g 3 (604)
4 degranulation (606)
5 abscess (608)

PART II

1 b, c, d (603)
2 b, c, d (603)
3 b, c, d (601, 611)
4 b, c, d (601)
5 b, c, d (603)
6 a, b (604)
7 a, b, c, d (606–607)
8 a, b, c, d (609)
9 a, c, d (611)
10 a (611–613)

CHAPTER 17 • MODULE II

PART I

1 IgG, IgA, IgM, IgD, IgE (615)
2 bone marrow (613)
3 antigens (613)
4 cytotoxic, helper, suppressor T cells (614)
5 hypersensitivity (629)
6 natural killer (624)

PART II

1 c, d (614–615)
2 a, b, c, d (618–619)
3 a, d (620–621)
4 a, b, c, d (621–623)
5 b (623)
6 b, c, d (624–625)
7 b, c, d (626–627)
8 a, c (627)
9 b (629–630)
10 a, b, c, d (630)

CHAPTER 17 • MODULE III

1 a, b, c, d (633–634)
2 a, b, d (634)
3 a, b, c, d (633–634)
4 b (634–635)
5 a, b, c (635)
6 b, c, d (635)

CHAPTER 17 • MODULE IV

PART I

1 Secretion of cortisol and activity of the sympathetic nervous system are usually increased. (636)
2 pharmacological effects (639)
3 See figure 17-25, page 637

PART II

1 a (638)
2 b, c, d (639.)
3 b, c, d, e (639)
4 a, b, d (639–640)

18
THE SENSORY SYSTEMS

Module I • Sensory neural pathways and somatic sensation
Module II • Vision
Module II • Hearing, vestibular system, and chemical senses
Module IV • Further perceptual processing

Module I • Sensory neural pathways and somatic sensation

OBJECTIVES

Upon completion of this module, the student will be able to:

1 Differentiate between *afferent information* and *sensory information.*
2 Define *perception.*
3 Describe the function of *specific* and *nonspecific pathways.*
4 Differentiate between *primary sensory cortex* and *somatosensory cortex.*
5 Define *polymodal neuron.*
6 Describe the general ascending pathway for somatic sensation.
7 Describe the size and site of cortical representation of somatic sensation.
8 Differentiate among the receptor systems for touch-pressure, joint position, temperature, and pain.
9 Differentiate between rapidly adapting and slowly adapting mechanoreceptors.
10 Define *proprioception.*
11 Define *kinesthesia.*
12 Define *nociceptors.*
13 Describe the role of *substance P, serotonin, norepinephrine, GABA, enkephalin,* and *endorphin* on the perception and response to pain.

READING ASSIGNMENT

Chap. 18, pp. 641–647.

EXERCISES

Directions: Answer the questions in the space provided.

1 By giving examples, highlight the differences in afferent information, sensory information, and the perception of a stimulus. **641**

2 Describe the pathway from somatic receptors to the sensory cortex. **642–644**

3 Describe the relationship between the size of the somatosensory cortex and the areas of the body with greatest sensitivity. **644**

4 Why is deep visceral pain more difficult to localize than a pinprick on a fingertip? **646**

5 Explain why the same painful stimulus can be perceived very differently by the same individual. Use the concept of descending pathway inhibition. **646–647**

SELF-TEST

PART I

Directions: Circle the correct answer(s).

1 Which of the following best describes a specific pathway?
 a A single neuron and all the receptor units that innervate it.
 b Parallel chains of interneurons that are grouped together.
 c One that indicates only that something is happening, not what or where.
 d Afferent neurons and interneurons themselves inhibit other parallel afferent components.
 e Several sensory units converge on a given chain of neurons that respond to the same stimulus energy.
 f A chain of three to five synaptically connected neuronal links.

2 A pacinian corpuscle is a receptor for which of the following?
 a temperature b pain c joint position d touch-pressure changes

3 Receptors signaling joint position are activated by which of the following stimuli?
 a light pressure on the skin of the arm
 b stretching to take a book off a high shelf
 c twisting or rotating the arm as in turning a door knob
 d normal movements such as walking
 e no movements at all
 f painful movements such as those felt by most people trying to touch their wrist with their thumb

4 The stimuli that give rise to pain result in which of the following?
 a sensory experience
 b reaction including emotional and behavioral responses
 c neither of the above

5 Which of the following are true regarding the pain sensory system?
 a Two ascending pathways to the brain are probably used simultaneously.
 b The pathway to the cerebral cortex conveys information about the pain, which is poorly localized and duller than that which goes to the reticular formation and thalamus.
 c The pathway to the brainstem reticular formation is involved in perception of the pain stimulus.
 d Receptors fire more rapidly as the stimulus severity increases.
 e The specific pathway ascends to the thalamus and the cerebral cortex.
 f Descending pathways can alter the transmission of information in afferent neurons.

PART II

Directions: Circle T for true and F for false.

T F 1 By receptor, we mean the afferent-nerve fiber ending or the specialized receptor cell associated with it.

T F 2 The pacinian corpuscle signals pressure.

T F 3 All joint receptors fire faster in extension than in flexion.

T F 4 Specific temperature-sensitive corpuscles respond to the full range of biologically compatible temperatures.

T F 5 Cold receptors increase their rate of discharge when cooled.

T F 6 The sensation of pain cannot be separated from the emotional and behavioral reaction.

T F 7 All afferent information coming to the central nervous system is called sensory information.

T F 8 The somatosensory cortex of the brain contains fibers subserving the sensory modalities of touch, temperature, taste, sight, and hearing.

Module II • Vision

OBJECTIVES

Upon completion of this module, the student will be able to:

1 Describe in general terms that part of the electromagnetic spectrum that is known to stimulate the receptors of the eye.
2 Describe the general structure of the eye using the following terms: *retina, optic nerve, fovea, iris, vitreous humor, aqueous humor, lens, pupil, cornea*, and *ciliary muscles.*
3 Define *accommodation* and describe its role in focusing an image on the retina.
4 Define *presbyopia, cataract, myopic vision, hyperopic vision*, and *astigmatism*, and the defect that is responsible for each.
5 Describe the role of the iris in regulating the amount of light entering the eye.
6 Describe the general structure of the *rod cell.*
7 Contrast the properties of rod and *cone* vision.
8 Differentiate between the functioning of the *rods* and *cones* and describe the role of each in visual acuity and dark adaptation.
9 List the elements of the visual pathway in order of processing visual information.
10 Describe the relationships among receptive fields and the *simple, complex*, and *hypercomplex* cells of the visual cortex.
11 Describe color vision and the basis of color-defective vision.
12 Describe the two basic types of eye movement and describe the adaptive value of each.

READING ASSIGNMENT

Chap. 18, pp. 647–657.

EXERCISES

Directions: Answer the following questions in the space provided.

655–656 1 Why does a blue sky look blue and not green? (Describe in terms of light receptor function.)

648 2 What does the lens of the eye do in the process of accommodation?

649 3 Accommodation is (easier/more difficult) ____________________ in older people. Why?

652–653, 657 4 Which of the two types of visual receptor cell is responsible for dark vision, visual acuity, color perception, and brightness? Describe the importance of the fovea in this aspect of vision.

652 5 Show the order of elements of the visual pathway by filling in the spaces in Fig. W-27 (see Fig.18-13, p. 652).

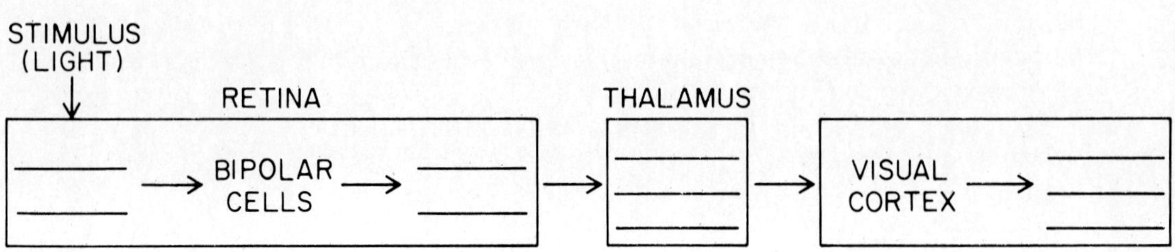

Fig. W-27

6 State the configuration of receptive fields to which the simple and the complex cells are sensitive. 654

____

____

____

SELF-TEST

PART I

Directions: Circle T for true and F for false.

T F 1 The entire electromagnetic spectrum is detected by the eye.
T F 2 The change in shape of the cornea to focus the visual image is called accommodation.
T F 3 Both the cornea and the lens function to focus the visual image on the retina.
T F 4 Visual acuity in dim light is due in part to the shift from rod to cone receptors.
T F 5 The visual system does not form a picture in the brain, but, through the simultaneous activation of many neurons, it forms a specifically coded electrical statement.
T F 6 Cortical cells of the primary visual cortex may be classified as either simple or complex according to the stimuli to which they respond.

PART II

Directions: Fill in the blanks as indicated.

1 The process of changing the shape of the lens to adjust for distance in focusing the visual image on the retina is called ______________________.

2 Match the items in column A with those in column B. Answers may be used more than once.

Column A	Column B
I _____ sometimes referred to as a nearsighted eye	a farsighted
II _____ sometimes referred to as a farsighted eye	b nearsighted
III _____ far objects focused in front of the retina	c myopic
IV _____ near objects focused behind the retina	d hyperopic
V _____ irregularities in the cornea	e astigmatism
	f cataract
	g accommodation
	h retina

VI ______ can be corrected or compensated for by eyeglasses

VII ______ results when the eyeball is too long for the lens

VIII ______ results when the eyeball is too short for the lens

3 The following are statements describing rod and/or cone receptor cells of the eye. Indicate whether the statement describes a rod (R), a cone (C) or both (R,C).

I ______ contain light-sensitive molecules called photopigments

II ______ are most numerous in the fovea

III ______ act as photoreceptors during conditions of poor illumination and for night vision

IV ______ have very high visual acuity

V ______ indicate or respond to brightness

VI ______ indicate color

VII ______ synapses on a bipolar cell

4 Arrange the following items in the proper order (from 1 to 7) to show the processing of visual information.

I ______ visual cortex

II ______ ganglion cells

III ______ stimulus

IV ______ rods and cones

V ______ visual association cortex

VI ______ lateral geniculate nucleus

VII ______ bipolar cells

5 The ______________________ cells are arranged to provide information about lines and borders.

6 The ______________________ cells are sensitive to corners or tongue-shaped objects.

7 The three cell types in the visual cortex are ______________________, ______________________, and ______________________.

8 What are the two types of eye movement?

a ______________________

b ______________________

9 What is the wavelength portion of the electromagnetic spectrum to which the receptors of the eye are sensitive? ________________

10 Simple cells of the primary visual cortex have receptive fields that are
a concentric on-off, i.e., circular.
b side by side with straight boundaries.
c sensitive only to a moving stimulus.

Module III • Hearing, vestibular system, and chemical senses

OBJECTIVES

Upon completion of this module, the student will be able to:

1 Define *frequency, amplitude*, and *purity* in relation to the reception of sound by the ear.
2 Describe the transmission of sound from the atmosphere to the *oval window*, including the role of each structure in the outer and middle ear.
3 Describe the role of the *oval window, basilar membrane, scala vestibuli, scala tympani, hair cells, organ of Corti, tectorial membrane*, and the *best frequency* in the reception of sound.
4 Describe the *place principle.*
5 Describe the basic structural elements of the *vestibular system* and their role in detection of motion and position.
6 Describe the receptor mechanisms for *taste* and *smell.*

READING ASSIGNMENT

Chap. 18, pp. 657–669.

EXERCISES

Directions: Answer the following questions in the space provided.

1 Explain why a person could not be heard talking in a perfect vacuum. 657

____

____

____

657–658 2 Explain what is meant by a "pure" tone.

____

____

____

657 3 What is the difference between frequency and amplitude of a sound?

____

____

____

4 The cells that generate impulses corresponding to sounds coming into the ear are called ______________________. Describe the mechanism of how
663 they function.

____

____

____

5 What part of the basilar membrane responds to high-pitch sounds? Low-pitch
662 sounds?

____

____

____

6 Why is the force per unit area on the oval window 15 to 20 times greater than
660 that on the tympanic membrane?

____

____

____

7 The two main functions of the vestibular system are to ______________ and to ______________________. These functions are performed by structures known respectively as the ______________________ and the
663–664 ______________________ and ______________________

8 The system for sensing taste can differentiate both quality and quantity. Explain
667–668 how these differ in terms of firing of action potentials of specific taste receptors.

____

____

____

9 Explain the difference in sensitivity and discrimination capability between taste and smell receptor cells. 667–669

____

____

____

SELF-TEST

PART I

Directions: Fill in the blanks as indicated.

1 Match the following.

	Column A	Column B
I ______	loudness of a sound	a purity
II ______	number of sound frequencies in addition to the fundamental tone	b frequency
III ______	related to the pitch of the sound	c amplitude

2 Match the structure of the ear with its function.

	Column A	Column B
I ______	transfers movements of the air in the outer ear to the fluid-filled chambers of the inner ear	a oval window
II ______	couples the tympanic membrane with the oval window	b cochlea
III ______	transmits sound (pressure) waves to the tympanic membrane	c ear canal
IV ______	separates the middle and inner ear	d middle-ear bones
V ______	senses sound waves coming through the ear canal	e eustachian tube
		f tympanic membrane

3 Choose the proper sequence of events (from 1 to 7) in the transmission of sound through the middle and inner ear.

I ______ The region of maximal displacement of the basilar membrane varies with the frequency of vibration of the sound source.

II _______ Where the displacement of the basilar membrane is a maximum, the stimulation of the hair cell receptors that ride on the membrane is the greatest.

III _______ The pressure wave passes up the ear canal and pushes in on the tympanic membrane.

IV _______ A wave of pressure is produced in the scala vestibuli on the inner-ear side of the oval window.

V _______ Most of the pressure waves are transmitted to the basilar membrane, which is deflected into the scala tympani.

VI _______ The chain of bones rocks the foot plate of the stapes against the oval window, causing it to bow into the inner ear.

VII _______ In normal hearing the greater potentials formed by the activated cells lead ultimately to the production of action potentials in the peripheral endings of the afferent nerves, the resulting action potentials being transmitted to the central nervous system.

4 The sounds heard most keenly by human ears are those from sources vibrating at frequencies between _______________ and _______________, but the entire range of frequencies audible to human beings extends from _______________ to _______________.

5 The vestibular system contains mechanoreceptors specialized to detect changes in _______________ and _______________.

6 Match the following.

	Column A	Column B
I _______	semicircular canals	a rate of change of motion of head
II _______	utricle and saccule	b provides information about the position of the head relative to the direction of the forces of gravity

PART II

Directions: circle the correct answer(s).

1 Which of the following are structures of the inner ear?

a stapes
b scala vestibuli
c scala tympani
d eustachian tube
e tectorial membrane
f cochlea
g basilar membrane
h hair cells
i tympanic membrane

2 Which of the following are true for the basilar membrane?
   a magnifies the sound impulse
   b sorts out incoming sound waves along its length
   c supports sound receptors called hair cells
   d is associated with a structure called the tectorial membrane
   e is more elastic closer to the oval window
   f divides the cochlea into the scala vestibuli and the scala tympani

3 Which of the following are true for hearing?
   a Because sound must travel through the air, a sound on the left stimulates the left ear before it stimulates the right ear.
   b When there are no air molecules, as in a vacuum, there can be no sound.
   c The human ear can detect differences in both frequency and amplitude of sounds.

4 Which of the following are true of the vestibular apparatus?
   a detects direction of sound
   b is a membranous sac
   c is in the temporal bone of the skull
   d contains three semicircular canals
   e contains hair cells that vibrate faster with louder sound input
   f contains a slight bulge for the utricle and saccule
   g contains endolymph

5 Which of the following are correct for taste reception?
   a Quality of taste is transmitted by the frequency of action potentials from receptor cells.
   b Individual molecules of a chemical substance bind with specific sites on the receptor cell membrane.
   c The chemical substance–receptor site combination alters the cell membrane potential.
   d The membrane of the receptor cell depolarizes when the cell is stimulated chemically.
   e Quantity of taste is related to variation of relative sensitivity of receptor cells in a group of neurons.

6 Olfactory discrimination depends on which of the following?
   a action potential pattern generated in the different afferent neurons
   b histological appearance of the receptor cell
   c head congestion in the nasal passages
   d physical alertness
   e patency of the eustachian tube
   f hunger
   g sex
   h smoking
   i heart rate above 100 beats/min

PART III

Directions: Circle T for true and F for false.

T F 1 The pressure on the tympanic membrane is the same as that on the oval window for the same impulse.

T F 2 Most sound impulses passing through the oval window travel the full length of the scala vestibuli, then pass into the scala tympani.

T F 3 Sound impulses passing from the scala vestibuli into the scala tympani without being transmitted by the basilar membrane are likely to be of low pitch rather than high pitch.

T F 4 Otoliths are tiny calcium carbonate stones found only in the endolymph fluid of the semicircular canals.

T F 5 The hair cells of the semicircular canals are stimulated only during changes in rate of motion.

T F 6 The utricle and saccule contain the receptors of the vestibular system that provide information about the position of the head relative to the direction of the forces of gravity.

T F 7 Current theory relating to taste sensation states that there are separate and distinct cells for each of the basic taste sensations, and action potentials are fired when a chemical substance related to that basic category contacts the cell.

T F 8 The frequency of action potentials in single nerve fibers of the taste system increases in response to increasing concentrations of the chemical stimulant.

T F 9 Awareness of a specific taste of a substance probably depends on the relative activity in a number of different neurons rather than that in a specific neuron.

T F 10 Receptor mechanisms for smell are probably differentiated at the chemical substance–receptor site level.

T F 11 The olfactory cells are differentiated into basic groups for specific odor sensations, as are those for taste.

Module IV • Further perceptual processing

OBJECTIVES

Upon completion of this module, the student will be able to:

1 Differentiate between the roles of the somatosensory and *cortical association areas* of the cortex in the process of perception.
2 List and describe four factors known to distort our perception.
3 Differentiate between *perception* and *sensory input.*
4 Differentiate between *false information* received by a receptor and a *perceptual illusion.*

READING ASSIGNMENT

Chap. 18, pp. 669–670.

EXERCISES

PART I

Directions: Fill in the blanks as indicated.

1 Match the following. **669–670**

I ______ required for complex integration
II ______ required for basic sensory input
III ______ connects primary cortical sensory or motor areas
IV ______ elaborates sensory information

a somatosensory cortex
b association area

2 List four factors known to distort our perception. **670**

a ______________________________
b ______________________________
c ______________________________
d ______________________________

3 Match the following. **669–670**

I ______ brain's analysis of events
II ______ information obtained at receptor level
III ______ modified by many factors
IV ______ always a conscious event
V ______ has many levels

a sensory input
b perception

PART II

Directions: Is there a difference in perception at the cortical level between false information (such as electric stimulation of a receptor) and a perceptual illusion? Explain. **669–670**

____
____
____

SELF-TEST

PART I

Directions: Fill in the blanks as indicated.

1 A part of the brain that, when lost, results in the loss of a specific sense (e.g., sight) is known as ______________________.

2 That part of the brain that is able to add further elaboration to a basic sense and is of great importance in the maintenance of higher mental activities is called a(n) ______________________.

3 Indicate by entering an A or an S whether the statement describes the association cortex (A) or the somatosensory cortex (S).

I ______ Permits logical interpretation of perceptions.

II ______ Loss of this part of the brain results in the loss of a specific modality.

III ______ Allows information processing for appropriateness.

IV ______ Compares information received by one sensory modality with that of another sensory modality.

V ______ Is of great importance in maintenance of higher mental activities.

4 Match the following:

a false information
b perceptual illusion

I ______ Contrary to our perceptual learning.

II ______ Damage to the receptor.

III ______ Action potentials in a given afferent pathway going to a certain area of the brain signal the kind of information normally carried in the pathway (i.e., stimulus can be in the form of electric or action potential).

IV ______ Can be proved false by physical measurements.

V ______ Occurs at the receptor level.

VI ______ Occurs at the cortical level, i.e., does not fit previous pattern.

PART II

Directions: Circle the correct answer(s).

Which of the following describe factors known to distort our perceptions?

a afferent information distorted by receptor mechanisms and by afferent information processing along afferent pathways

b loss of the somatosensory cortex
c emotions, personality, and social background
d lack of suitable receptors for many energy forms
e information entering the central nervous system but not giving rise to conscious sensations

Answers

CHAPTER 18 • MODULE I

PART I

1 e (642)
2 d (644–645)
3 b, c, d, e, f (645)
4 a, b (646)
5 a, d, e, f (646–647)

PART II

1 T (643)
2 F Signals changes in pressure. (644–645)
3 F There is a mixture, i.e., some fire this way, and some do just the opposite. (645)
4 F (645–646)
5 T (645)
6 F This can be done by drugs or operation on the brain, interrupting pathways connecting the frontal lobe of the cerebrum with other brain parts. (647)
7 F Sensory information is only that segment of the total afferent input that has a conscious correlate, i.e., a conscious awareness of the physical world. (641)
8 F Sight, hearing, and possibly taste are not represented in the somatosensory cortex. (642)

CHAPTER 18 • MODULE II

PART I

1 F Only a small portion, between 400 and 700 nm. (647)
2 F Lens changes shape. (648)
3 T (648)
4 F (652)
5 T (653–654)
6 T (654)

PART II

1 accommodation (648)
2 I c (650)
II d (650)
III b, c (650)
IV a, d (650)
V e (650)
VI a, b, c, d, e (650)
VII b, c (650)
VIII a, d (650)
3 I R, C (651)
II C (657)
III R (652)
IV C (652)
V R (652)
VI C (651)
VII R, C (652)
4 I 6
II 4
III 1
IV 2
V 7
VI 5
VII 3 (652)
5 simple cortical (655)
6 hypercomplex (655)
7 simple, complex, hypercomplex (654)
8 a fast (saccades) (657)
b slow (tracking) (657)
9 400–700 nm (647)
10 b (655)

CHAPTER 18 • MODULE III

PART I

1 I c (657)
II a (658)
III b (657)
2 I d (659)
II d (659)
III c (658)
IV a (659)
V f (658)
3 I 5 (662)
II 6 (663)
III 1 (658)
IV 3 (660–661)
V 4 (662)
VI 2 (659)
VII 7 (663)
4 1000; 4000 Hz; 20; 20,000 Hz (657)
5 motion, position of head(663)
6 I a (666)
II b (666)

PART II

1 b, c, e, f, g, h (660–662)
2 b, c, d, f (662–663)
3 a, b, c (657)
4 b, c, d, f, g (663–666)
5 b, c, d (667–668)
6 a, c, d, f, g, h (668–669)

PART III

1 F (660)
2 F (662)
3 T (662)
4 F (666)
5 T (665)
6 T (666)
7 F (667)

8 T (667)
9 T (668)
10 T (668)
11 F (668)

CHAPTER 18 • MODULE IV

PART I

1 primary (visual) cortex or somatosensory cortex (669)
2 cortical association cortex or areas (669)
3 I A (669)
II S (669)
III A (669)
IV A (669)
V A (669)
4 I b (670)
II a (670)
III a (670)
IV b (670)
V a (670)
VI b (670)

PART II

a, b, c, d, e (669–670)

19

CONTROL OF BODY MOVEMENT

Module I • Local control of motor neurons
Module II • Descending pathways, posture, balance, and walking

Module I • Local control of motor neurons

OBJECTIVES

Upon completion of this module, the student will be able to:

1 Define *motor unit* and the *motor neuron pool.*
2 List the three basic types of motor units.
3 Define *movement program.*
4 Name the two descending pathways from cortical neurons to spinal cord motor neurons.
5 List three characteristics of *voluntary* motor activity.
6 Differentiate between voluntary and involuntary motor activities and state the role of learning in the development of involuntary responses.
7 Describe the *monosynaptic stretch reflex* by identifying each component in both anatomical terms and as elements of a negative-feedback control system for muscle length.
8 Define *polysynaptic reflex.*
9 Describe the role of *reciprocal innervation* and activation of synergistic muscles in the knee jerk.
10 Differentiate between *synergistic* and *antagonistic* muscles.

11 Differentiate between *alpha* and *gamma motor neurons.*
12 Define and describe the significance of *alpha-gamma coactivation.*
13 Describe a *Golgi tendon organ* and state its function.
14 Describe the *crossed-extensor reflex.*
15 Define *interneurons* and describe their functions.

READING ASSIGNMENT

Chap. 19, pp. 671–679.

EXERCISES

PART I

Directions: Answer the following questions in the space provided.

673–675 1 Defend or refute the statement "Involuntary activity is nothing more than monosynaptic and polysynaptic reflexes strung together."

____

____

____

674–678 2 Since synergistic and antagonistic muscles have opposite actions why would they be involved simultaneously in limb movement?

____

____

____

678 3 Describe the function of the Golgi tendon organ.

____

____

____

PART II

Directions: Diagram a monosynaptic reflex in Fig. W-28. Use the symbols suggested. The only known monosynaptic reflex is the stretch reflex. Your answer should match A on Fig. 19-5, p. 677.

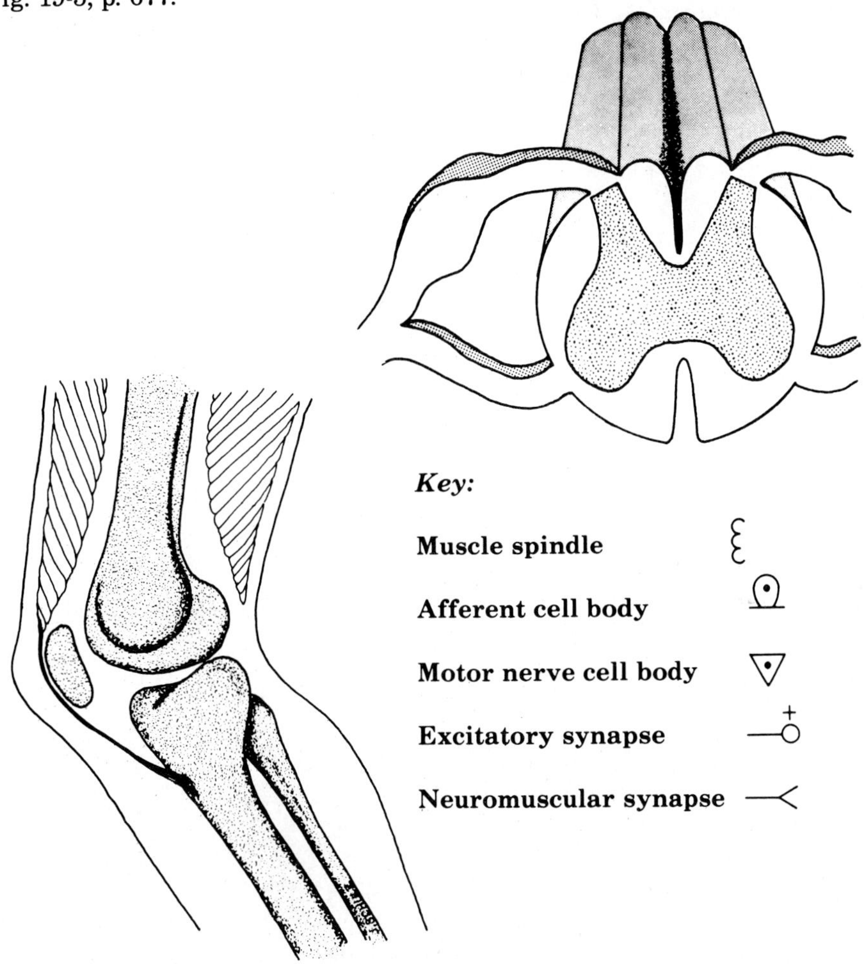

Fig. W-28: Monosynaptic reflex.

SELF-TEST

PART I

Directions: Circle the correct answer(s).

1 Contraction of a skeletal muscle
  - a increases tension of the spindle stretch receptors.
  - b increases the firing rate of afferent neurons leaving the muscle spindle.
  - c increases the tension on the Golgi tendon organs.
  - d increases the firing rate of afferent neurons leaving the Golgi tendon organ.

2 Which of the following structures are involved in alpha-gamma coactivation?
 a spindle muscle fiber
 b gamma motor neuron
 c alpha motor neuron
 d Golgi tendon organs

3 Almost all motor behavior
 a involves a conscious component.
 b involves an unconscious component.
 c is purely voluntary.
 d is purely involuntary.

4 The crossed-extensor reflex
 a is a monosynaptic reflex.
 b is a strictly voluntary response.
 c causes the same action in the opposite limb.
 d causes the opposite response on the other side of the body.
 e is a polysynaptic response.

PART II

Directions: Complete the following items in the space provided.

1 The excitation of one muscle and the simultaneous inhibition of its antagonistic muscle is called ______________________________.

2 The motor neurons controlling the skeletomotor muscle fibers are classified as ______________________________.

3 Axons of what type of motor neurons innervate the spindle fibers? ______________________________.

PART III

Directions: Circle T for true and F for false

T F 1 The motor neurons that activate the spindle fibers are the same motor neurons that activate the skeletomotor muscle fibers.

T F 2 The gamma motor neurons are activated primarily by synaptic input from descending pathways.

T F 3 The selection of the specific pattern of neural activity is the function of centers in the spinal cord.

T F 4 The knee jerk is a good example of a negative-feedback control system.

T F 5 Stretch reflexes are the only known polysynaptic reflex arcs in man.

Module II • Descending pathways, posture, balance, and walking

OBJECTIVES

Upon completion of this module, the student will be able to:

1 Describe three mechanisms by which descending pathways modify the activity of alpha motor neurons.
2 Differentiate between the direct corticospinal (*pyramidal*) pathway and the multineuronal (*extrapyramidal*) pathway in both anatomical and functional terms.
3 Describe the interactions of the *motor cortex*, the *premotor area*, and *subcortical centers* in relation to coordination of muscle movement.
4 Differentiate between the *readiness potential* and the *motor potential*.
5 Diagram the neural loops connecting the cortex, thalamus, basal ganglia, and the motor neuron.
6 Describe the neural deficit in persons with *Parkinson's* disease.
7 Differentiate between the role of cortical input and general afferent input in the overall functioning of the cerebellum.
8 List the four general defects in movement that are associated with cerebellar damage.
9 List one or more examples of the five components of the reflex arc that would be involved in the maintenance of posture and balance.
10 Define *proprioceptors*.
11 Define *central pattern generator* and describe its role in walking.

READING ASSIGMENT

Chap. 19, pp. 679–689.

EXERCISES

PART I

Directions: Answer the following questions in the space provided.

You have a patient who was in an accident that resulted in some cerebellar damage. Keeping this in mind, answer the following questions.

1 How does the cerebellum affect the motor activity? **685–686**

____

____

____

686 2 Does destruction of the cerebellum cause loss of any specific movement?

686 3 What kinds of problems might this patient suffer from?

PART II

Directions: Answer the following questions in the space provided.

The mutineuronal pathway is a kind of descending pathway by which the cerebral cortex, subcortical centers, and cerebellum influence the motor neurons.

1 Draw a simple diagram of the multineuronal pathway (see Fig. 19-9, p. 681).

2 What kind of information does this pathway transmit?

3 Does the information that is transmitted by this pathway change or stay the same as it goes down through the cerebrum and brainstem? Why?

4 Is the multineuronal pathway functionally separated from the direct corticospinal pathway? How does that change its function?

PART III

Directions: Complete the following chart by giving the name of the correct part of the brain corresponding to the different properties.

Properties	Name of the Part of the Brain
Origin of descending pathways to motor neurons	____________________ **679–680**
Control of postural mechanisms, coordination of the simultaneous movements of locomotion	____________________ **685–686**
Voluntary control of slow smooth movements	____________________ **680–681**
Influences the parts of the brain responsible for motor activity	____________________ **684–685**

SELF-TEST

PART I

Directions: Circle the correct answer(s).

1 The fibers of the direct corticospinal pathway end on
  a alpha motor neurons. c gamma motor neurons.
  b beta motor neurons. d interneurons.
2 The multineuronal motor pathway descending from the cortex synapses in the
  a basal ganglia. c cerebellum.
  b brainstem nuclei. d dorsal root ganglia.
3 The afferent inputs to the cerebellum come from which of the following?
  a eyes b skin c nose d joints
4 The postural reflexes occur whenever a person is
  a sitting. c rocking on a rocking chair.
  b walking on a rope. d falling.

PART II

Directions: Answer the following questions in the space provided.

1 What are the five components of the reflex arc?

  a ____________________

  b ____________________

  c ____________________

d ______________________________

e ______________________________

2 Because of its shape in some parts of the brain, the direct corticospinal pathway is called ______________________________ or ______________________________.

3 When a person with cerebellar damage tries to move the limbs, he or she goes into ______________________________ or ______________________________.

PART III

Directions: Circle T for true and F for false.

T F 1 The skeletal muscles on the left side of the body are controlled largely by neurons in the left half of the brain.

T F 2 The direct corticospinal pathway is the major mediator of fine movements.

T F 3 The basal ganglia serve a special role in influencing the voluntary control of sustained motor behaviors.

Answers

CHAPTER 19 • MODULE I

PART I

1 c, d (676–678)
2 a, b, c (677–678)
3 a, b (674)
4 d, e (679)

PART II

1 reciprocal innervation (677)
2 alpha motor neurons (677)
3 gamma motor neurons (677)

PART III

1 F They are not the same; gamma innervates spindles and alpha innervates skeletomotor. (677)
2 T (677)
3 F Higher brain centers. (672)
4 T (676)
5 F Monosynaptic. (676)

CHAPTER 19 • MODULE II

PART I

1 a, c, d (681)
2 a, b, c (681)
3 a, b, d (686)
4 a, b, c, d (686–688)

PART II

1 a receptor
b afferent pathway
c integrating center (CNS)
d efferent pathway
e effector (157)
2 pyramidal tract, pyramidal system (680)
3 to-and-fro tremor, oscillation (686)

PART III

1 F In the right half of the brain. (680)
2 T (680-681)
3 T (684-685)

20
CONSCIOUSNESS AND BEHAVIOR

Module I • Consciousness
Module II • Behavior

Module I • Consciousness

OBJECTIVES

Upon completion of this module, the student will be able to:

1 Define *states of consciousness* and distinguish this from *conscious experience.*
2 Describe the basis of the *electroencephalogram* (*EEG*).
3 Define *alpha rhythm* and describe the range of oscillation frequencies and the subjective mood often associated with it.
4 Define the *beta rhythm* and *EEG arousal* and describe the range of oscillation frequencies and the subjective mood often associated with it.
5 Compare *slow wave sleep* with *paradoxical sleep* (or *REM sleep*) in terms of EEG pattern, duration, ease of arousal, muscle tone, cardiovascular and respiratory state, and episodes of dreams.
6 Describe the role of the *reticular formation* in controlling states of consciousness.
7 Describe the two opposing systems for maintaining arousal or sleep.
8 Describe the role of *serotonin, delta sleep-inducing peptide* (*DSIP*), and *substance S* in sleep.
9 Define *directed response, orienting response, habituation,* and *dishabituation.*
10 Describe the postulated role of the *locus ceruleus* in directed attention.
11 Describe the role of sensory input in the maintenance of normal conscious experience.

READING ASSIGNMENT

Chap. 20, pp. 690–697.

EXERCISES

PART I

Directions: Draw the EEG patterns (indicating time and voltage) associated with the following states of consciousness or rhythms; describe the subjective sensation asso-
691–692 ciated with each.

1 alpha rhythm

2 beta rhythm

3 slow wave sleep

4 paradoxical sleep

PART II

Directions: States of consciousness are also identified by their behavioral aspects. Put an X in the appropriate spots of the following chart to indicate that a behavior is
691–692 present in the state of consciousness listed.

Behavior	Alert	REM Sleep	Slow Wave Sleep
Eyes open			
Eyes closed and relaxed			
Tonus in postural muscles			
Lack of tonus in postural muscles			
Irregular change in respiration and heart rate			
Easy to arouse			
Difficult to arouse			
Dreaming			

PART III

Directions: Define the following terms.

1 states of consciousness ______________________________

____

2 conscious experience ______________________________

____

3 orienting response ______________________________

____

4 dishabituation ______________________________

____

5 habituation ______________________________

____

6 novelty detectors ______________________________

____

SELF-TEST

Directions: Circle the correct answer(s).

1 During slow wave sleep
a the sleeper can be awakened easily.
b dreams are more likely to occur than during paradoxical sleep.

c muscle tone is inhibited.
d respiration and heart rate are regular.

2 During paradoxical sleep
a there are periodic episodes of rapid eye movements.
b blood pressure is variable.
c the EEG waves are slower and larger than in slow wave sleep.
d the EEG pattern looks similar to that during the alert state.

3 Which of the following statements are true concerning neural mechanisms for directed attention?
a The term *directed attention* refers to the process of dishabituation.
b An orienting response is a *behavior* directed toward the stimulus source.
c Activity of neurons in the locus ceruleus increases with the end of REM sleep.
d Activity of neurons in the locus ceruleus increases with increased sensory stimulation.

4 Which of the following statements are correct concerning sleep?
a Release of serotonin from the raphe nuclei is thought to induce sleep.
b The peptide DSIP has been implicated in inducing paradoxical sleep.
c Substance S has been shown to induce slow wave sleep.
d The only known function for the reticular formation is the control of sleep-wake cycles.

Module II • Behavior

OBJECTIVES

Upon completion of this module, the student will be able to:

1 Define *motivation.*
2 Describe *reward* and *punishment* in behavioral terms.
3 Describe *self-stimulation* experiments and the conclusions drawn from them.
4 Describe the brain areas involved in motivated behavior.
5 List the chemical transmitters known to be involved in motivation.
6 Describe the two ways of characterizing emotions.
7 Describe the relationship between the limbic system and emotion.
8 Define *schizophrenia;* describe the various hypotheses concerning the causes of schizophrenia.
9 Define *depression, mania,* and *bipolar affective disorder;* describe the various hypotheses concerning the causes of these disorders.
10 Define *psychoactive drug.*
11 Define *tolerance* to a drug.

12 List possible causes for drug tolerance.
13 Describe the theory behind the physical symptoms associated with *withdrawal.*
14 Define *addiction.*
15 Describe the effects of alcohol on the central nervous system.
16 Define *coma.*
17 List the criteria used to determine *brain death.*
18 Describe the *chemoaffinity theory* of nerve-connection development.
19 List three general factors that influence neural organization.
20 Describe the role of adequate nutrition and hormones in brain development.
21 Define *cretinism.*
22 State the role of the *critical period* in neural development.
23 Define *memory* and *memory trace.*
24 Compare *short-term memory* with *long-term memory*, including a discussion of *memory consolidation.*
25 Contrast *procedural* (*verbal*) with *declarative* (*nonverbal*) memories.
26 Describe the various theories of the neural basis of learning and memory.
27 Define *retrograde amnesia.*
28 Define *plasticity* in the nervous system.
29 State the role of the left cerebral hemisphere in language function.
30 Distinguish between *Broca's area* and *Wernicke's area* in the formulation of language.
31 Describe the functions of the right cerebral hemisphere.
32 Define *aphasia.*

READING ASSIGNMENT

Chap. 20, pp. 697–715.

EXERCISES

PART I

Directions: In self-stimulation experiments, electric stimuli are delivered to specific parts of the brain through an implanted electrode. The results of such studies add to the knowledge of functions of particular areas of the brain. With this in mind, answer the following questions.

1 Is increased self-stimulation of a brain area punishing? ______________________ **698–699**

____

2 Are stimuli to some areas of the hypothalamus rewarding? ______________________

____

3 What indicates that this is so? ______________________

____

4 What areas of the brain are most closely related to highly rewarding self-stimulation? ______

______

5 Which important pathway carries information between the brainstem and limbic area and is implicated as an area involved in motivated behaviors? ______

______

PART II

Directions: Answer the following questions in the space provided.

700–701 1 Describe the relationship between the hypothalamus and the limbic system in respect to their involvement in emotion.

______

______

______

709 2 Adequate nutrition and hormones have an important role in brain development. Give an example to show the effect of decreased hormones during development.

______

______

______

709–710 3 John wanted to get the phone number of the graduate school. He looked up the number in the directory, shut the directory, and dialed the number.

a What type of memory is this? ______

b Are procedural memories or declarative memories involved in this process?

______

c Is there an exclusive site for memory storage? ______

d Does the removal of some parts of the brain remove specific memories? ______

______

707 4 List five criteria frequently accepted for establishing "brain death."

a ______

______

b ______

______

c ____

____

d ____

____

e ____

____

5 A patient has been taking a drug for weeks and finds that the dose must be increased to give the same effect. What might be the cause of this? **703**

____

____

____

6 A patient suffers from symptoms that you diagnose as drug withdrawal. You are convinced that this patient is addicted to a specific drug. Explain what addiction is, and outline the current thinking concerning the cause of withdrawal to this patient. **704–705**

____

____

____

7 Describe the role played by Broca's area and Wernicke's area in speech. **713–714**

____

____

____

SELF-TEST

PART I

Directions: Complete the following statements.

1 In a self-stimulation experiment if the animal increases its bar-pressing rate above control, the electric stimulation is assumed to be ______________________

2 A fragmentation of mental functioning is known as ______________________.

3 Swings between manias and depressions are known as ______________________.

4 ______________________ to a drug occurs when increasing doses of that drug are required to achieve effects that initially occurred in response to smaller doses.

5 The physical symptoms associated with cessation of a drug use are known as ______________________.

6 According to the ______________________ theory, neural circuits are said to grow and organize themselves according to selective attractions between neurons, which are determined by chemical codes under genetic control.

7 The memory that exists during the time a memory trace is being laid down is called ______________________.

8 Retrograde amnesia following unconciousness does not affect ______________________ memory.

9 The ability of neural tissue to change its responsiveness to stimulation because of its past history of activation is known as ______________________.

10 A language deficit in an individual who is neither retarded nor has paralysis of the muscles involved in speech is known as ______________________.

PART II

Directions: Circle the correct answer(s).

1 The following drugs may affect motivation:
  a amphetamines.
  b dopamine.
  c norepinephrine.
  d chlorpromazine.

2 Schizophrenia
  a affects approximately 10 percent of the population.
  b simply means a swing between mania and depression.
  c may be caused by excessive activity of dopamine-mediated synapses in the limbic system.
  d is basically the same as bipolar affective disorders.

3 Tolerance to a drug
  a occurs when a drug causes increased effects with decreasing dosages.
  b may be caused by an increase in degradative-enzyme concentration in the liver.
  c may occur as a result of feedback mechanisms decreasing the release of the naturally occurring transmitter.
  d can only affect drugs that act on the limbic system.

4 Criteria for "brain death" include
  a unconsciousness, but the ability to respond to loud noises.
  b breathing, but only with difficulty.
  c flat EEG.
  d an absence of cortical and brainstem reflexes.
  e an increase in brain–blood flow for a period of at least 30 min.

5 According to the chemoaffinity theory of neural development,
  a certain neurons are attracted to each other.
  b during early development, neurons are capable of chemically identifying each other.
  c the precision of neural connections leads to highly specific synaptic connections.
  d the control of neural growth and development is entirely dependent on the genetic code; environmental influences are unimportant.

6 Experiments that have located "rewarding" areas in the brain and that use implanted electrodes are called
  a split-brain experiments.
  b self-stimulation experiments.
  c neurosurgical experiments.
  d electrode experiments.

7 A person with a severe deficit in declarative memory may experience the following:
  a an inability to learn new motor skills.
  b a loss of nonverbal memory.
  c an inability to remember what has happened.
  d a deficit in short-term memory.

8 The following hormones and drugs have been shown to alter ability to learn and retain information:
  a epinephrine.
  b endorphin.
  c ACTH.
  d enkephalin.

9 The language area in the temporal lobe is called
  a Kluger's area.
  b Broca's area.
  c Wernicke's area.
  d D'Alecy's area.

10 Damage to Broca's area will result in
  a expressive aphasias.
  b an inability to understand spoken language.
  c little speech deficit if this occurs before 2 years of age.
  d little speech deficit if this occurs before early adulthood.

Answers

CHAPTER 20 • MODULE I

PART I

1 a, d	(692)
2 a, b, d	(692)
3 b, c, d	(694–695)
4 a, c	(693–694)

CHAPTER 20 • MODULE II

PART I

1 rewarding	(698)
2 schizophrenia	(701)
3 bipolar affective disorders	(702)
4 tolerance	(703)
5 withdrawal	(704)
6 chemoaffinity	(708)

7 short-term memory (710)
8 long-term memory (711)
9 plasticity (712)
10 aphasia (715)

PART II

1 a, b, c, d (699–700)
2 c (701–702)
3 b, c (703)
4 c, d (707)
5 a, b, c (708–709)
6 b (698)
7 c (710)
8 a, b, c, d (711–712)
9 c (713)
10 a, c (715)

NOTES

NOTES

NOTES

NOTES

NOTES

NOTES

NOTES

NOTES

NOTES

NOTES